Meal Prep

Beginners Guide to Clean Eating Meal Prep – Includes Recipes to Give You Over 50 Days of Prepared Meals!

by Olivia Rogers

Copyright © 2018 By Olivia Rogers
All rights reserved. No part of this book may be reproduced in any form without permission in writing from the author. No part of this publication may be reproduced or transmitted in any form or by any means, mechanic, electronic, photocopying, recording, by any storage or retrieval system, or transmitted by email without the permission in writing from the author and publisher.
For information regarding permissions write to author at Olivia@TheMenuAtHome.com
Reviewers may quote brief passages in review.

Please note that credit for the images used in this book go to the respective owners. You can view this at: TheMenuAtHome.com/image-list

Olivia Rogers
TheMenuAtHome.com

Table of Contents

Who Is This Book For? _____ 6

What Will This Book Teach You? _____ 7

Introduction _____ 8

Chapter 1: Understanding Clean Eating in Meal Prep _____ 10

Chapter 2: Benefits of Prep Meal Planning _____ 13

Chapter 3: Getting Started _____ 16

Chapter 4: Additional Tips for Better Meal Prepping _____ 20

Chapter 5: Refilling Your Pantry _____ 23

Chapter 6: 50-Day Prep Meal Plan _____ 25

Blueberry Waffles _____ 36

Smoked Tofu and Vegetable Sushi Roll _____ 37

Peanut Butter and Strawberry Jam Quinoa Bowl _____ 38

Cinnamon Zucchini Muffin _____ 40

Edamame Pate Sandwiches _____ 42

Savory Dutch Baby Pancake _____ 44

Muffin-Tin Quiches with Smoked Cheddar and Potato ____ 46

Avocado-Egg Sandwich _____ 48

Lemony Linguine with Spring Vegetables _____ 49

Banana Bran Muffins _____ 51

Tuscan Bean and Kale Stew _____ 53

Burmese Chicken _____ 55

Squash and Red Lentil Curry _____ 57

Poached Cod and Green Lentil Beans with Pesto _____ 59

Mexican Chicken Avocado Salad _____ 61

Parsley & Garlic Chicken Cutlets with Broccoli	63
Low-Carb Mexican Casserole	65
Spiced Tempeh Tacos with Creamy Cashew Sauce	67
Crispy Fried Salmon with Spring Vegetable Broth	69
Fish Sticks	71
Salisbury Steak with Mushroom Gravy	73
Southwestern Turkey Quinoa Stuffed Peppers	75
Swedish Meatballs	77
Shrimp Ceviche and Avocado Salad	79
Cauliflower Risotto with Seared Scallops	81
Mac & Cheese with Collards	83
Mini Pepperoni Pizza	85
Steak Skewers with Strawberry Chimichurri	86
Freezer Beans and Cheese Burritos	88
Spaghetti with Quick Meat Sauce	90
Peanut Butter-Oat Energy Balls	92
Mango Fruit Leather	93
Peanut Butter Banana Cups	95
Apple Nachos	96
Fried Shallots	97
Homemade Pesto Sauce	98
Clean Eating Ranch Dressing	99
Aioli	100
Caramel Sauce	101
Clean Eating Peanut Butter	102
Garlic-Parmesan Popcorn	103

Homemade Cherry Pie Bars	*105*
Quince Crumble Bars	*106*
Pumpkin Candied Popcorn	*108*
Clean Eating Pumpkin Pie Spice	*109*
Clean Eating Breakfast Cookies	*110*
Apple Peanut Butter Sandwich	*112*
Honey Nut Granola	*113*
Buffalo Hummus	*115*
Healthy Energy Bites	*116*
Mayonnaise-less Avocado & Greek Yogurt Tuna Salad	*117*
Pumpkin Spice Overnight Oats	*119*
Conclusion	*120*
Final Words	*121*
Disclaimer	*123*

Who Is This Book For?

Are you a busy career person, housewife, student or anyone who is constantly on the go?

When you are busy with the daily routine that leaves you no time to prepare healthy food to suit your physical activities and stay healthy, then this book is truly made for you.

The book hopes to cater to people who need or want to have a healthy diet but got no options to benefit from a clean eating meal because of their hectic schedule.

When you are constantly on the go and everything for you seems to be in a constant rush, meal prep could be the best solution to your needs.

This way of preparing the meal is extremely popular especially for office employees, working moms, construction workers, road drivers, students, and even people actively involved in the fitness industry. It helps fitness enthusiasts and athletes stay on a steady, healthy diet. With meal prep, you can have a heathy diet prepared in less time. While it keeps your diet on track, it likewise helps you save on your pocket.

What Will This Book Teach You?

It's hard to keep away from unhealthy but convenient options like fast foods and ready-to-eat-meal packs along with instant foods that one usually finds in a grocery store. It's obvious that the jet-set lifestyle that most of us live today is the top reason that barred us from clean eating as according to a study conducted by the American Journal of Health.

However, if you intend to keep yourself and your family healthy, it is a must to integrate clean eating into your lifestyle. But how can you do this?

Meal prep is the best solution for this issue. When you don't have enough time for preparing meals, then you can always plan ahead and be time-efficient. Managing your time in preparing meals also equates to saving on your food budget.

This book is geared towards accomplishing this goal of saving time and money on a clean eating diet.

Furthermore, this book will teach you many things that are essentials to healthy eating and among them are the following

- How to plan ahead for your meal preparation.
- How to choose foods that are essentially healthy.
- How to prepare easy-to-cook healthy meals on the budget.
- How to shift to a healthier lifestyle.

Introduction

As many are gaining awareness on the importance of clean eating and living a healthy lifestyle, many are trying to cope with the difficulties of preparing meals. The availability of time and the temptations that surround us in forms of unhealthy processed foods along with the rampant existence of food chains serve as a mounting struggle that keeps us from shifting to the right direction.

When time is significant in achieving your health goal, then you need to do some planning to keep up with it and there's no better way to do it better than by doing it in the kitchen through the meal prep method.

What is Meal Prep?

It's either you've heard about meal prep or you haven't heard at all. If you belong to those you haven't encountered the term before, then let's discuss it a little further.

In a meal prep, you cook one big meal and divide it into several packs to last for a whole 5-working days or even a week. The primary reason for this is you don't have to rush every morning to prepare for your breakfast or lunch and dinner when you have to work all day and go home fully exhausted. Neither would you have to prepare daily but rather prepare it in advance, seal it in a clean container, and store it in the refrigerator to make it available when you need them.

As many are gaining awareness on the importance of clean eating and living a healthy lifestyle, many are trying to cope with the difficulties of preparing meals.

When time is significant in achieving your health goal, then you need to do some planning to keep up with time and there's no better way to do it better in the kitchen than by meal prep method.

With the industrial revolution, people are migrating to the cities where opportunities are great compared to the countryside. Along with it is coping with the hustle-bustle lifestyle in the city. As speed became a significant element in your everyday living, your lifestyle becomes a mixture of routine activities, rush periods, and instant meals.

This type of lifestyle endangered everyone with unhealthy habits giving rise to major illnesses including obesity, diabetes, hypertension, leaky gut, and other health issues.

This jet-set style of living likewise causes you too much stress which is also pointed out as the number one health risk factor in many of these death-leading illnesses. Unless people will shift to a healthy lifestyle, they will be subject to constant health threats.

Coping with stress and other health risk factors involves a radical shift. Adopting Clean Eating is a lifestyle and not just a passing fad. Before you submit to this, make sure that you have the determination and commitment to integrate it into your life along with your family.

Unless you are living alone, the whole family needs to be involved in it. Even kids need to be educated on the clean eating diet and when they are big enough to help you, then you exposed and involved them in meal prep planning. This will ensure that you are not alone in your advocacy.

Since the whole family is involved in eating, educate everyone on what you are doing or supposed to do. The younger the children are taught about Clean eating meal prep, the easier it will be integrated into their consciousness. Once they get into the habit, it will automatically grow in them and they can easily adjust to the immediate shift in lifestyle.

It would be more beneficial if you let the children help you in the kitchen. You can also ask for suggestions from them. Never underestimate a child's ability to create ideas when you ran out of them as children's creativity is always on the go and they are showing more creativity than us.

Chapter 1: Understanding Clean Eating in Meal Prep

Treating clean eating as a lifestyle rather than a diet is the bottom line for understanding Clean Eating. You don't have to embrace clean eating for the simple reason that you want to lose weight or just because it's trending. Clean eating is making a choice of what you want to eat to stay healthy - either you take those junks in or out of your life.

Clean Eating is Awareness

Clean eating doesn't mean that you have to eat everything raw. It simply means choosing minimally processed food and being aware of its contents. Reading the label before purchasing a product is typically part of the awareness.

The more localized the product, especially farm and agricultural products, the more these are considered safe and clean over those products that are highly processed and manufactured.

Scanning the item's label can be as significant as searching for harmful ingredients in foods that you eat. Make sure, therefore, that the label bears a list of ingredients that you can easily recognize and avoid additive content like artificial flavoring and coloring.

Cooking Clean is Going Back to the Basics

Going back to the very basics is the essence of clean eating - may it be in cooking, choosing of ingredients or preserving leftovers.

It's quite right to say that nutrients like Vitamin C are lost when cooked which makes it necessary for them be consumed raw. However, there are nutrients like lycopene that is more potent when cooked. Therefore, it's best to eat a wide variety of foods in both forms - raw and cooked.

When cooking, avoid the use of high fat including deep frying and stewing in either animal or vegetable fats. Rather opt for stir-frying and steaming. Take note, however, steaming is just a second option in terms of preserving the nutritional value of the food. As much as possible, fruits and vegetables are best eaten raw.

Selecting organic foods are always preferable to avoid taking in added substance and hormones that are sometimes present in foods and are hazardous to the human body.

Clean Eating is Knowing When it is Enough

Clean eating does not provide you a free leeway to eating more than what is necessary in terms of quantity. These foods are healthy, but they still have calories in them that eating in large quantity may have a reversed effect on your body.

It is for this reason that meal prep greatly complements clean eating and maximizes its efficiency.

An owner of a seasonally influenced café in New York City suggests that when eating clean, think of your plate as divisible by five. One portion for food rich in protein, one portion for healthy carbohydrates, and the remaining three portions are allocated to fruits and veggies.

Now, that you have understood the concept of Clean Eating, it's time that we integrate this into our meal preparation process.

Meal prepping is a convenient way of preparing your food when you don't have much time to cover the conventional type of meal preparation and cooking aside from being cost-effective.

Read This FIRST - 100% FREE BONUS

FOR A LIMITED TIME ONLY – Get Olivia's best-selling book *"The #1 Cookbook: Over 170+ of the Most Popular Recipes Across 7 Different Cuisines!"* absolutely FREE!

Readers have absolutely loved this book because of the wide variety of recipes. It is highly recommended you check these recipes out and see what you can add to your home menu!

Once again, as a big thank-you for downloading this book, I'd like to offer it to you *100% FREE for a LIMITED TIME ONLY!*

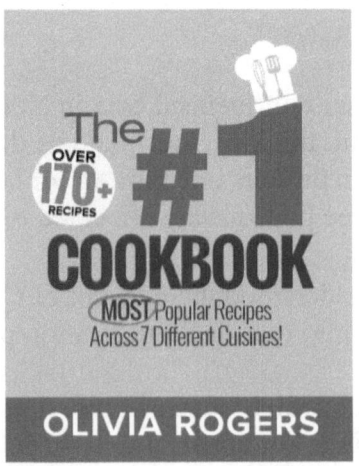

Get your free copy at:

TheMenuAtHome.com/Bonus

Chapter 2: Benefits of Prep Meal Planning

When it comes to a dietary shift, meal planning can make a big difference. It would be easy to cook a quick convenience food when everything in your kitchen is planned and well-organized.

The Benefits of Meal Planning

Meal planning is significant to healthy eating and there are many ways you can benefit from meal planning. Even if you're a veteran in healthy eating, meal preparation and cooking can take much of your time if you don't practice meal planning, so I encourage you to take half an hour every week to plan clean healthy meals for the family.

Benefits of Prep Meal Planning include the following:

- **A Cut in Your Budget**

    Food takes a great portion of our family budget and stretching it can make an impact on the overall budget. In times when financial matters arise that forces us to tighten our budget, preparing meal would be more difficult. You may still be eating solid food but still, you have to focus on providing nourishing food for the family. With meal prep planning, you can be able to have both benefits.

- **Eat Real Food**

    Consuming a well-planned real food diet is likewise vital in many aspects of our health. To do this, you need to have some real advance planning. Meal planning allows you to decide the kind of healthy food you will be purchasing before going to the grocery store. With this, you don't need to spend more on foods you would not actually be using for the week.

    When you are switching to a healthier diet, it makes meal planning essentially more important to make everyone stick to a healthy lifestyle as you start learning the ropes.

- **Avoid Food Wastage**

    One of the significant issues that one faces in the kitchen are finding containers of food pushed back to the inside of the fridge and realizing that they have been there for weeks or months – long enough to make them appear like a science experiment.

    If you are considering healthy lifestyle, then you might as well include learning how to be a good steward of the resources you have. With proper planning, you are making sure that supplies and ingredients are used within a week and nothing more. You should not throw away any leftovers just because you were not able to consume them within a week. Meal planning makes it possible for you to use your creativity to the max, so you can avoid wastage.

- **Less Stress**

    Every health enthusiast is aware that stress is the culprit to every illness. It is indeed stressful when you have to stay eating at night and wake up very early in the morning, so you can prepare for your family meals. This stress is even more doubled when you have more worries in the workplace that worrying over your means is the east among them.

    Regardless of what you are doing, someone had to prepare the meals and you know it's not that easy. It's time-consuming and tedious, not to count the time and effort you have to spend in selecting items including reading labels and identifying what's clean and not clean. However, if you plan in advance and do some cooking in advance, then you won't have to worry about what to eat for the week. Effective planning in whatever you do lessens the stress and save you much time and energy.

- **Save Time**

Another great benefit you can get from Meal Prep planning is the fact that it helps you save an enormous amount of time. If you spend an hour in the kitchen for morning preparation, another 30 minutes for noon break and another 30 minutes for dinner, it means you are spending at least one and a half hour a day or 10 hours and a half in a week of 7 days. In a month's time, you are saving more than 3 days of meal preparation time if you have a meal plan.

When you can plan ahead, you can cook in bulk and store it properly for future meals. You can also make some extra protein bars for snacks in case you want to take something healthy with you on your sports game, in class or workplace.

In the winter, you may make use of slow cooker meals and store it in the freezer then stick one in the crockpot on busy days.

- **Add Variety**

It's easy to think that my planning is boring, but based on statistics, there are more families that are eating the same meals over and over again in the absence of a meal plan. With the advance planning, you can ensure variety in your meals and avoid eating the same food on the same day.

When it comes to a dietary shift, meal planning can make a big difference. It would be easy to cook a quick-convenience food when everything in your kitchen is planned and well-organized.

Chapter 3: Getting Started

Getting started is not easy with meal prep. It could sound confusing at first but once you get acquainted with the technique, everything would just flow smoothly. You may create your own template for the diet plan you have for the week.

To get started, here are steps that will guide you through the process.

Plan Ahead

When you start making your plan, consider the number of meals you need to prepare for the whole week. You can either plan for 5 days if you intend to cook regular meals during Saturdays and Sundays. Figure out what meals you have to prepare as you need to consider factors like events, dates that involve eating out, travel, and other things that would affect your meal plan.

Proper planning will help you avoid wasting food and save money.

Schedule Your Prep Day

You may be too busy on workdays, so you have to schedule your prep day on weekends. In scheduling, you must consider the availability of your foods and other materials that you may need on that particular day. When you start preparing your meal, you can't waste your time going back to the grocery store to buy something that you missed just because you haven't check it out previously. Always remember that time is of the essence in meal prep.

Before going to the grocery store and purchasing your supplies, ingredients, and materials, make sure that you are done with your meal planning. You have likewise determined your 5-Day Meal Plan or One-Week Plan. Most do their food shopping on Saturday and prep meals on Sunday. But there are others who meal prep on Sunday and Wednesday depending on the need based on the number of people who would be consuming them.

Some people buy foods and ingredients online, but people who are into clean eating meals prefer to buy through suppliers nearest to them to be assured of the freshness and quality.

Select Your Menu

When you have determined how many meals you would be preparing for the week, then it's time to choose what you would eat in the days ahead. In choosing your meals, keep these in mind.

"Meals Need to be Nutritious and Well-Balanced."

As you select the kind of food to eat in every meal, aim for 30-40 grams of protein, 50-60 grams of carbohydrates, and 15-20 grams of fat.

Involve Creativity!

Prepping ingredients in large quantity is much easier than cooking in small amounts. However, eating the same stuff over and over is quite boring, so you have to find ways to use basic ingredients in different ways.

Like for instance, you can cut beef sirloin into cubes for beef stew, julienne cut for stir-fries or simply roast or grill it like steak. You can eat carrots, cucumber raw or with dip, or have these stir-fried.

Utilize Leftovers

When you just can't avoid having leftovers because of sudden occasion or event, do something about your leftovers. Don't simply throw them away. You can either reheat or make a new recipe out of it.

Why do you have to use leftovers?

Based on the National Resources Defense Council estimates, about 40 percent of food grown, processed, and transported to the United States is never consumed.

Likewise, the Food and Agriculture Organization of the United Nations reported that roughly 70 billion of food is lost annually in the U.S. alone and about one-third of that food waste happened because people purchase, cook or serve more than what is actually needed while one in every six Americans goes hungry according to Feeding America.

Getting into the habit of throwing away leftovers is impacting this significant global issue.

It Helps Lose Weight

With health issues everywhere, more and more people are getting aware of their health status and tantamount to that is their weight. When obesity seems to be common or associated with death-leading diseases, many are finding ways to lose weight effectively – food intake, exercises, medication.

Many diets are introduced – Vegan, Paleo, Ketogenic, Mediterranean, etc. All their methods are helpful but not applicable to all. Many take each method like a sprint and shifted from one to another. They tend to forget the fact that to acquire your ideal weight, you need to fully embed it into your lifestyle.

By adopting Clean Eating Meal Prep, you are consolidating two significant methods in weight loss – e.g., regulating food quantity and quality.

Planning your meals can do a lot to help you in your weight loss goal as you can limit the amount of food that you will consume based on your daily requirement. With a weekly meal prep routine, it allows you full control on how many calories you have to consume daily which can be a perfect recipe for weight loss.

It Creates in You Healthy Habits

As you get used to Clean Eating Prep Meals, you realized the importance of eating the proper way for your body to get the most benefits from foods you are consuming.

Healthy eating habits include choosing nutrient-pack meals instead of unhealthy junk food you usually find in a food chain, choosing quality over quantity or enhancing your knowledge of clean foods, and proper way of preparing meals that can provide you with maximum benefits at the most reasonable cost.

Chapter 4: Additional Tips for Better Meal Prepping

Storage

Food storage is vital for every meal prepping activity. It will save you time, energy, and money if you are preparing just enough for what you will need in the coming week. Proper refrigeration and freezing are essential steps for a successful planning.

However, there is always this possibility that some food hiding in a drawer or the farthest corner of your refrigerator will be forgotten for too long making it spoiled and wasted. Don't forget to able your food on the date they were prepared so you can track when to use them. In storing, make sure that attest prep meals are paced at the back with the oldest meals right there on the front row.

Store highly perishable items – leafy vegetables, herbs, greens, and chopped fruits at eye level and occupying the front and center part of the storage area.

In freezing, there are foods that worked better than others. When kept in airtight containers, cooked meals freeze well and those high in moisture content like green salads, watermelons, and tomatoes become mushy and thawed. Try a little blanching before freezing can help but when the texture of the frozen foods appears to be undesirable, you can use them in soups or stews.

Here are recommended times for different cooked foods that offer the best flavor with maximum nutrients content and food safety.

Freezing at 0°F or lower

- 2-3 months: Cooked beans, soups, and stews 3-6 months: Poultry and cooked or ground meat
- 6-8 months: Chopped fruit (apples, banana, pears, mango, and plums) and berries stored in a freezer bag

- 8-12 months: Vegetables, if blanched first for about 3-5 minutes (depending on the vegetable)

Refrigeration at 40°F or lower

- 1-2 days: Cooked ground beef or ground poultry
- 3-4 days: Cooked whole meats, poultry, and fish; stews and soups
- 5 days: hummus, cooked beans;
- 1 week: chopped vegetables if stored in an air-tight container, hard-boiled eggs
- 2 weeks: Cheese (soft and opened)
- 5-6 weeks: Cheese (hard and opened)

Once you have the system in place, planning won't be that hard. However, there are some things you have to keep in mind when starting out.

Focus on Favorite Recipes

After a few weeks of trying the Prep Meal, you can spot some recipes that you and your family would love to eat. Try to keep about 20 of these recipes on your list and you won't be ever bored with your meal again. This way, it would be easier for the whole family to stick to a healthy-eating lifestyle.

Each week, you use each of these favorite recipes for five on your dinners. You may try some new dinner recipes on weekends. You can also build your list to something in season to take advantage of seasonal products which are much cheaper when they are in season. In a clean eating, local produce is suggested than purchasing them via sources you don't know. Doing this will help you save more on the budget.

Your Protein

Protein can be the most expensive part of every meal that if you can make use of less expensive cuts and stretch them, it might allow you to buy organic meats rather than the farm-bred types. With brews and casseroles, you can add more veggies and stretch more of the meat compared to when you're serving baked or roasted meat. Using your slow cooker can be a great way to tenderized tougher meats that are usually cheaper.

Mix It Up with Spices

It could be surprising how you can create a variety of meals by just changing the spices. A basic Chicken Squash Stir Fry Recipe can have a Mexican taste by simply adding cumin and chili powder. If you want the Indian taste, add some curry.

For Italian flavor, basil, thyme, oregano, and garlic are frequently used. If you prefer your meal to have an Asian flair, use the popular Chinathat 5 spices.

Don't Be A Short Order Cook

Are your kids a bunch of picky eaters? It's probably because they can eat what they want, and you prepare food that caters to their preferences only rather than complements to their dietary requirements.

Exposing your children to healthy and diverse foods while they're young prevents them from having food preferences. Most children don't like eating green and leafy vegetables, but if they're used to it, they will gladly take whatever there is that is offered before them. It's not only that healthy eating will make them strong. Some foods can likewise affect their moods and responses. So, you raise happier kids when teaching them to eat a healthy diet.

Chapter 5: Refilling Your Pantry

In refilling your pantry, bear in mind that you will be using ingredients that are clean foods.

So, what are clean foods?

Clean foods are those that are closest to their natural state – meaning, they are minimally processed and therefore retained more of their nutrients.

Unprocessed Foods

- Farm fresh eggs
- Dried legumes
- Nuts
- Fresh fruits and vegetables

Minimally Processed

- Frozen fruits and vegetables
- Unprocessed meat from wild and grass-fed animals
- Hormone-free dairy
- Unrefined grains including bread, brown rice, quinoa, pasta, steel-cut oatmeal, and popcorn
- Oils

Take Inventory of Your Stocks

Before you start meal prepping, make sure that your inventory of supplies and materials is in ready. So better start checking in your pantry. Take note of what you will need and list them down on your shopping list before rushing out to the grocery store. Check on every item and make sure that everything on the menu you will be preparing are there on your shopping list.

Stock on Staples

Stock your pantry with a variety of reliable supplies including dried herbs, spice blends, and whole grains. Don't forget to add foods you frequently used in cooking like olive oil, garlic, onions, etc. This will simplify meal prepping. Staple foods best complement meal prep menu.

Make a Round-Ups of Your Containers

Containers are an essential part of meal prepping and depending on your plans for the week, you will be needing an assortment of containers for storage including glass and plastic bottles, zipped bags that can be stored in a freezer, and containers for packed lunches. If you are watching your weight, it's recommended that you pack meal-prep foods in containers in recommended sizes, so you don't exceed your limit for the quantity of food you need to consume.

Chapter 6: 50-Day Prep Meal Plan

Now, that you have decided to start with meal prepping clean foods which is a fit and healthy lifestyle, you have to prepare your Diet Meal Plan. But how much should you eat?

In preparing your diet plan, you don't need to be obsessed with macros or counting calories. Healthy-eating means stress-free and taking track of what goes into your body as you eat is even more stressful.

However, healthy eating and watching your portions is a good point to start. We usually eat 5-6 meals in a day and this must be a balanced meal of lean protein, healthy fats, and carbs, with a lot of vegetables. Don't forget fruits as well.

Since you will be prepping food in advance, you can easily watch over your recommended portions by putting just enough food with the recommended size in your container.

We are giving you here a general guideline on daily recommendations while you are still starting. Do keep in mind, however, that shifting to a new lifestyle is a continuing process and not a just trend-based fad. Everybody is made differently, and you know your body more than anyone else. This is a continuing trial-and-error process until you find out what works best for you.

- Fat – around 0.5 gram per pound of body weight.
- Carbohydrates – around 1.0 gram per pound of body weight.
- Protein – 1.0 gram {for weight-loss}-1.5 grams {for maintenance} per pound of body weight.
- Sugar – under 30 grams per day (keep your sugar derived mostly from fruit).

\multicolumn{6}{c}{**PREP MEAL DIET PLAN**}					
WEEK 1	**Monday**	**Tuesday**	**Wednesday**	**Thursday**	**Friday**
Breakfast	Mac and Cheese with Collards	Garlic Parmesan Popcorn	Tuscan Bean and Kale Stew	Mac and Cheese with Collards	Salisbury Steak with Mushroom Gravy And Green Salad
Snack	Garlic Parmesan Popcorn	Peanut Butter - Oats Energy Balls	Peanut Butter - Oats Energy Balls	Garlic Parmesan Popcorn	Garlic Parmesan Popcorn
Lunch	Tuscan Bean and Kale Stew	Salisbury Steak with Mushroom Gravy And Green Salad	Mac and Cheese with Collards	Tuscan Bean and Kale Stew	Salisbury Steak with Mushroom Gravy
Snack	Peanut Butter - Oats Energy Balls	Mac and Cheese with Collards	Garlic Parmesan Popcorn	Mac and Cheese with Collards	Garlic Parmesan Popcorn
Dinner	Salisbury Steak with Mushroom Gravy And Green Salad	Tuscan Bean and Kale Stew	Salisbury Steak with Mushroom Gravy And Green Salad	Peanut Butter - Oats Energy Balls	Tuscan Bean and Kale Stew

PREP MEAL DIET PLAN					
WEEK 2	Monday	Tuesday	Wednesday	Thursday	Friday
Breakfast	Southwestern Turkey Quinoa Stuffed Pepper	Smoked Tofu and Vegetable Sushi Roll	Burmese Chicken Salad	Smoked Tofu and Vegetable Sushi Roll	Peanut Butter Banana Cups
Snack	Peanut Butter Banana Cups	Peanut Butter Banana Cups	Southwestern Turkey Quinoa Stuffed Pepper	Mango Fruit Leather	Southwestern Turkey Quinoa Stuffed Pepper
Lunch	Burmese Chicken Salad	Mango Fruit Leather	Smoked Tofu and Vegetable Sushi Roll	Southwestern Turkey Quinoa Stuffed Pepper	Burmese Chicken Salad
Snack	Mango Fruit Leather	Southwestern Turkey Quinoa Stuffed Pepper	Mango Fruit Leather	Peanut Butter Banana Cups	Mango Fruit Leather
Dinner	Smoked Tofu and Vegetable Sushi Roll	Burmese Chicken Salad	Peanut Butter Banana Cups	Burmese Chicken Salad	Smoked Tofu and Vegetable Sushi Roll

PREP MEAL DIET PLAN					
WEEK 3	Monday	Tuesday	Wednesday	Thursday	Friday

Breakfast	Poached Cod and Green Lentil Beans with Pesto	Spaghetti with Quick Sauce	Squash and Red Lentil Curry	Poached Cod and Green Lentil Beans with Pesto	Spaghetti with Quick Sauce
Snack	Apple Nachos	Quince Bars	Apple Nachos	Quince Bars	Apple Nachos
Lunch	Squash and Red Lentil Curry	Poached Cod and Green Lentil Beans with Pesto	Spaghetti with Quick Sauce	Squash and Red Lentil Curry	Poached Cod and Green Lentil Beans with Pesto
Snack	Spaghetti with Quick Sauce	Apple Nachos	Quince Bars	Spaghetti with Quick Sauce	Quince Bars
Dinner	Quince Bars	Squash and Red Lentil Curry	Poached Cod and Green Lentil Beans with Pesto	Apple Nachos	Squash and Red Lentil Curry

PREP MEAL DIET PLAN					
WEEK 4	Monday	Tuesday	Wednesday	Thursday	Friday
Breakfast	Low-Carb Mexican Casserole	Edamame Pate Sandwich	Low-Carb Mexican Casserole	Edamame Pate Sandwich	Edamame Pate Sandwich

Snack	Edamame Pate Sandwich	Blueberry Waffles	Mexican Chicken Avocado Salad	Blueberry Waffles	Low-Carb Mexican Casserole Edamame Pate Sandwich
Lunch	Mexican Chicken Avocado Salad	Low-Carb Mexican Casserole	Pumpkin Candied Popcorn	Pumpkin Candied Popcorn	Mexican Chicken Avocado Salad
Snack	Blueberry Waffles	Pumpkin Candied Popcorn	Blueberry Waffles	Edamame Pate Sandwich	Pumpkin Candied Popcorn
Dinner	Low-Carb Mexican Casserole	Mexican Chicken Avocado Salad	Pumpkin Candied Popcorn	Mexican Chicken Avocado Salad	Blueberry Waffles

	PREP MEAL DIET PLAN				
WEEK 5	Monday	Tuesday	Wednesday	Thursday	Friday
Breakfast	Cauliflower Risotto with Seared Scallops	Parsley and Garlic Chicken Cutlets with Broccoli	Cauliflower Risotto with Seared Scallops	Parsley and Garlic Chicken Cutlets with Broccoli	Crispy Fried Salmon with Spring Vegetable Broth
Snack	Cookies	Cookies	Cinnamon Zucchini Muffins	Cauliflower Risotto with Seared Scallops	Cinnamon Zucchini Muffins

Lunch	Crispy Fried Salmon with Spring Vegetable Broth	Cauliflower Risotto with Seared Scallops	Parsley and Garlic Chicken Cutlets with Broccoli	Crispy Fried Salmon with Spring Vegetable Broth	Cauliflower Risotto with Seared Scallops
Snack	Cookies	Cinnamon Zucchini Muffins	Cookies	Cinnamon Zucchini Muffins	Cookies
Dinner	Parsley and Garlic Chicken Cutlets with Broccoli	Crispy Fried Salmon with Spring Vegetable Broth	Cauliflower Risotto with Seared Scallops	Crispy Fried Salmon with Spring Vegetable Broth	Parsley and Garlic Chicken Cutlets with Broccoli

	PREP MEAL DIET PLAN				
WEEK 6	Monday	Tuesday	Wednesday	Thursday	Friday
Breakfast	Banana Bran Muffins	Swedish Meatballs	Fish Sticks with Shredded Purple Cabbage and Lemon Wedge	Banana Bran Muffins	Swedish Meatballs
Snack	Muffin Tin Quiches with Smoked Cheddar and Potato	Banana Bran Muffins	Lemony Linguine with Spring Vegetables	Muffin Tin Quiches with Smoked Cheddar and Potato	Lemony Linguine with Spring Vegetables

Lunch	Swedish Meatballs	Fish Sticks with Shredded Purple Cabbage and Lemon Wedge	Swedish Meatballs	Lemony Linguine with Spring Vegetables	Fish Sticks with Shredded Purple Cabbage and Lemon Wedge
Snack	Muffin Tin Quiches with Smoked Cheddar and Potato	Lemony Linguine with Spring Vegetables	Banana Bran Muffins	Lemony Linguine with Spring Vegetables	Muffin Tin Quiches with Smoked Cheddar and Potato
Dinner	Fish Sticks with Shredded Purple Cabbage and Lemon Wedge	Swedish Meatballs	Muffin Tin Quiches with Smoked Cheddar and Potato	Fish Sticks with Shredded Purple Cabbage and Lemon Wedge	Banana Bran Muffins

PREP MEAL DIET PLAN					
WEEK 7	Monday	Tuesday	Wednesday	Thursday	Friday
Breakfast	Savory Dutch Pancake	Peanut Butter and Strawberry Jam Quinoa Bowl	Steak Skewers with Strawberry Chimichurri	Peanut Butter and Strawberry Jam Quinoa Bowl	Avocado - Egg Sandwich

Snack	Avocado - Egg Sandwich	Savory Dutch Pancake	Avocado - Egg Sandwich	Savory Dutch Pancake	Peanut Butter and Strawberry Jam Quinoa Bowl	
Lunch	Steak Skewers with Strawberry Chimichurri	Spiced Tempeh Tacos with Creamy Cashew Sauce	Peanut Butter and Strawberry Jam Quinoa Bowl	Steak Skewers with Strawberry Chimichurri	Spiced Tempeh Tacos with Creamy Cashew Sauce	
Snack	Savory Dutch Pancake	Avocado - Egg Sandwich	Spiced Tempeh Tacos with Creamy Cashew Sauce	Avocado - Egg Sandwich	Savory Dutch Pancake	
Dinner	Spiced Tempeh Tacos with Creamy Cashew Sauce	Steak Skewers with Strawberry Chimichurri	Avocado - Egg Sandwich	Peanut Butter and Strawberry Jam Quinoa Bowl	Steak Skewers with Strawberry Chimichurri	

PREP MEAL DIET PLAN					
WEEK 8	**Monday**	**Tuesday**	**Wednesday**	**Thursday**	**Friday**
Breakfast	Steak Skewers with Strawberry	Buffalo Hummus	Shrimp Ceviche and Avocado Salad	Steak Skewers with Strawberry	Spiced Tempeh Tacos

	Monday	Tuesday	Wednesday	Thursday	Friday
	Chimichurri			Chimichurri	
Snack	Mini Pepperoni Pizza	Mini Pepperoni Pizza	Spiced Tempeh Tacos	Buffalo Hummus	Mini Pepperoni Pizza
Lunch	Shrimp Ceviche and Avocado Salad	Spiced Tempeh Tacos	Buffalo Hummus	Shrimp Ceviche and Avocado Salad	Steak Skewers with Strawberry Chimichurri
Snack	Spiced Tempeh Tacos	Steak Skewers with Strawberry Chimichurri	Mini Pepperoni Pizza	Spiced Tempeh Tacos	Buffalo Hummus
Dinner	Buffalo Hummus	Shrimp Ceviche and Avocado Salad	Steak Skewers with Strawberry Chimichurri	Shrimp Ceviche and Avocado Salad	Mini Pepperoni Pizza

PREP MEAL DIET PLAN					
WEEK 9	Monday	Tuesday	Wednesday	Thursday	Friday
Breakfast	Freezer Beans and Cheese Burritos	Turkey Burger	White Bean Roasted Red Pepper	Avocado and Greek Yogurt Tuna Salad	Freezer Beans and Cheese Burritos

Snack	Turkey Burger	Energy Bite	Avocado and Greek Yogurt Tuna Salad	Energy Bite	Energy Bite
Lunch	White Bean Roasted Red Pepper	Freezer Beans and Cheese Burritos	Turkey Burger	White Bean Roasted Red Pepper	Avocado and Greek Yogurt Tuna Salad
Snack	Energy Bite	Avocado and Greek Yogurt Tuna Salad	Energy Bite	Freezer Beans and Cheese Burritos	Turkey Burger
Dinner	Avocado and Greek Yogurt Tuna Salad	White Bean Roasted Red Pepper	Freezer Beans and Cheese Burritos	Turkey Burger	White Bean Roasted Red Pepper

PREP MEAL DIET PLAN					
WEEK 10	**Monday**	**Tuesday**	**Wednesday**	**Thursday**	**Friday**
Breakfast	Garlic-Basil Shrimp with Zucchini Noodles	Pumpkin Spice Overnight Oats	Spinach and Broccoli Strata	Honey Nut Granola	Pumpkin Spice Overnight Oats
Snack	Honey Nut Granola	Spinach and	Homemade Cherry Pie Bars	Homemade Cherry Pie Bars	Garlic-Basil Shrimp

			Broccoli Strata			with Zucchini Noodles
Lunch	Pumpkin Spice Overnight Oats	Garlic-Basil Shrimp with Zucchini Noodles	Pumpkin Spice Overnight Oats	Spinach and Broccoli Strata	Honey Nut Granola
Snack	Honey Nut Granola	Homemade Cherry Pie Bars	Spinach and Broccoli Strata	Garlic-Basil Shrimp with Zucchini Noodles	Pumpkin Spice Overnight Oats
Dinner	Garlic-Basil Shrimp with Zucchini Noodles	Spinach and Broccoli Strata	Honey Nut Granola	Homemade Cherry Pie Bars	Spinach and Broccoli Strata

Blueberry Waffles

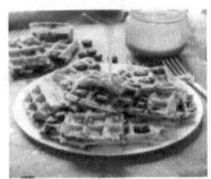

Servings: 5-6
Nutritional Information: Calories- 342; Fats- 20g; Carbohydrates- 36g; Protein- 10g

Ingredients

- ½ cup fresh blueberries
- 2 ripe bananas
- 3 large eggs
- 3 tbsp. plain and unsalted almond butter
- ½ tsp. pumpkin pie spice
- ½ tsp. pure vanilla extract
- ½ cup tapioca flour
- ¼ cup almond flour
- 2 tbsp. coconut oil

Directions

1. Preheat the waffle iron. Meanwhile, combine the bananas, almond flour, almond butter, tapioca flour, eggs, pumpkin pie spice, and vanilla extract in a blender and process until smooth. Transfer the batter to a bowl and fold in the blueberries.

2. Once the waffle iron is ready, brush some oil on the top and bottom of the iron. Put half a cup of batter to each waffle (for a 4-inch square) or 2/3 cup (for a 6-inch round). Repeat this step until all the batter is used. Let the waffles cool completely at room temperature. Store in an airtight container and freeze for up to 1 month.

Smoked Tofu and Vegetable Sushi Roll

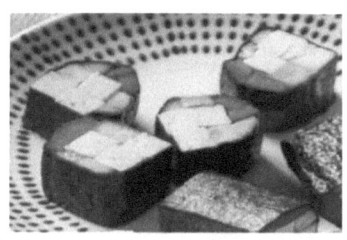

Servings: 5
Nutritional Information: Calories- 144; Fats- 7g; Carbohydrates- 8g; Protein- 7g

Ingredients

- 5 - 1 oz. organic baked smoked tofu, sliced
- 5 sheet nori, toasted
- 2 ripe avocados, sliced
- 6 cucumbers, cut into matchsticks
- 6 red bell peppers, thinly sliced

Directions

1. Place the nori with shiny-side down on a cutting board. Assemble the avocado, tofu, cucumber, and bell pepper end-to-end across the bottom third of the nori.

2. Carefully and tightly roll it up. Wet the last inch of the nori in order to seal the roll. Divide and cut into 8 pieces.

Peanut Butter and Strawberry Jam Quinoa Bowl

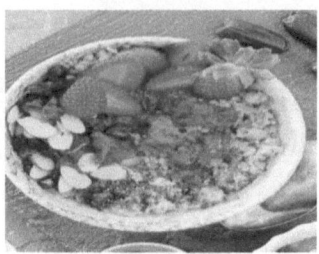

Servings: 5-6
Nutritional Information: Calories- 438; Fats- 17g; Carbohydrates- 63g; Protein- 13g

Ingredients

- 1½ cup quinoa
- 4 cups plain unsweetened almond milk (plus more for serving)
- 5 tbsp. peanut butter
- 2 ½ cup frozen strawberries, sliced
- 1 ½ tbsp. pure maple syrup
- 1½ tbsp. chia seeds
- 5 pitted dates, chopped
- 5 tbsp. almonds, chopped

Directions

1. Put a medium-sized saucepan over medium-high heat. Add the almond milk and quinoa. Bring it to a boil and stir in the peanut butter. Cover the pan with a lid and bring heat to low. Cook for another 13-15 minutes or until the quinoa is tender and the milk is absorbed. Remove the pan from the heat and keep the lid on.

2. While waiting for the quinoa mixture to boil, set another saucepan over medium-high heat, add the strawberries and

maple syrup. Cook for 7-9 minutes or until the strawberries release their juice and they begin to break down.

3. Using a fork, mash the berries. Add the chia seeds, reduce heat to low and continue to cook for another minute or two. Keep in mind to stir occasionally. Remove the pan from the heat and set it aside.

4. Fluff the quinoa with fork and divide between two storage containers. Top with strawberry mixture, almonds, and dates.

5. To serve, splash additional milk on top.

Cinnamon Zucchini Muffin

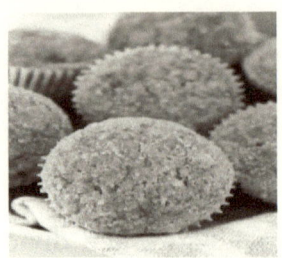

Servings: 10
Nutritional Information: Calories- 292; Fats- 11g; Carbohydrates- 43g; Protein- 5g

Ingredients

- 1 ¼ cups zucchini, finely shredded
- 1 ¼ cups whole-wheat pastry flour
- ½ cup pure maple syrup
- 1/3 cup ground flaxseeds
- 3/4 cup blanched almond flour
- ¼ cup coconut oil, melted
- 3/4 cup unsweetened raisins
- 1 tbsp. ground cinnamon
- 2 tsp. baking powder
- 1 tsp. baking soda
- ½ cup water
- ½ tsp. sea salt

Directions

1. Preheat oven to 350°. Line a muffin tray with 10 muffin liners. If there are empty slots, fill them halfway with warm water.

2. In a medium bowl, incorporate the flax seeds, almond flour, pastry flour, baking powder, baking soda, cinnamon, and salt.

3. In a large bowl, whisk the maple syrup, coconut oil, and water together. Add the dry ingredients and stir well. Gently fold the raisins and zucchini.

4. Pour the batter into the muffin tray slots with liners. Bake for 20-25 minutes. You can perform the toothpick test to check if they're done. Let them cool in the tray for about 5 minutes before transferring to the wire rack.

5. Remove the muffins from the tray and transfer them in a container. Store at room temperature (for three days) or freeze them (for up to 1 month).

Edamame Pate Sandwiches

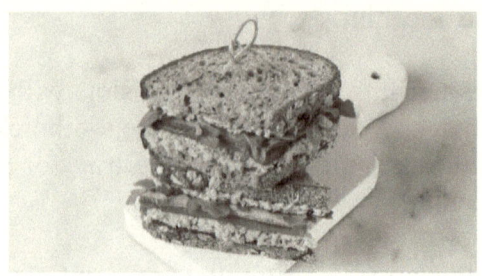

Servings: 5
Nutritional Information: Calories- 320; Fats- 15g; Carbohydrates- 35g; Protein- 14g

Ingredients

- 10 slices whole-grain bread
- 5 jarred roasted red peppers, drained and sliced
- 3 cups arugula
- 3 small cucumbers, thinly sliced
- 1 ½ cups frozen shelled organic edamame, thawed
- ½ cup raw unsalted walnuts
- 1/3 cup packed fresh mint leaves
- 1 green onion, chopped
- ½ tsp. sea salt
- 3 tbsp. fresh lemon juice
- 4 tbsp. water
- Extra-virgin olive oil, for drizzling

Directions

1. Put the walnuts, edamame, onion, mint, and salt in the food processor and process. With the motor running, add the water and lemon juice. Process until you achieve a smooth consistency.

2. Divide the pâté among the 5 bread slices. Also, divide the cucumber, pepper, and arugula among the 5 slices, putting them in layers. Drizzle with oil before topping them finally with the remaining slices.

Savory Dutch Baby Pancake

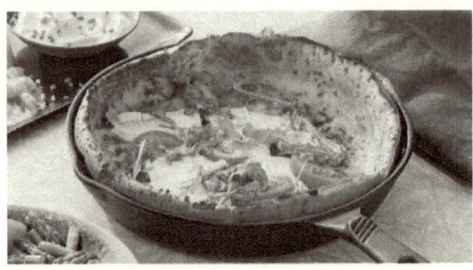

Servings: 5-6
Nutritional Information: Calories- 257; Fats- 15g; Carbohydrates- 19g; Protein- 11g

Ingredients

- 2 oz. Brie cheese, thinly sliced and cut into 1-inch pieces
- ½ cup white whole-wheat flour or whole-wheat pastry flour
- 2 Roma tomatoes, sliced
- 3/4 cup whole milk
- 2 tbsp. organic unsalted butter
- 3 large eggs
- 2 tbsp. fresh chives, chopped and divided
- ½ tsp. sea salt
- ¼ tsp. paprika
- ½ tsp. ground black pepper

Directions

1. Preheat oven to 425°. Process the flour, eggs, milk, paprika, pepper, and salt in a food processor for 2 minutes or until the mixture becomes light and fluffy. Remove the blade and let it stand for 15 minutes. Stir in 1 tbsp. of chives.

2. Melt butter in a 9-inch (or 10-inch) pan over medium-high heat until it starts foaming. Add the batter.

3. Bake it for about 18-20 minutes or until the pancake is puffed and browned.

4. Sprinkle Brie evenly on top of the pancake during the last minute of baking.

5. Carefully slide the pancake using a spatula onto a cutting board. Top it with tomato slices before garnishing it with the remaining chopped chives. Let it cool completely before storing in the fridge.

Muffin-Tin Quiches with Smoked Cheddar and Potato

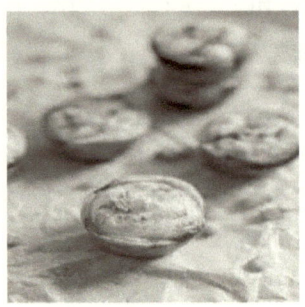

Servings: 6
Nutritional Information: Calories-238; Fats- 16g; Carbohydrates- 11g; Protein- 14g

Ingredients

- 1½ cups fresh spinach, chopped
- 1 cup smoked Cheddar cheese, shredded
- 1½ cups red-skinned potatoes, finely diced
- ½ cup low-fat milk
- 8 large eggs
- 1 cup red onion, diced
- 2 tbsp. extra-virgin olive oil
- ½ tsp. ground black pepper
- ¾ teaspoon salt, divided

Directions

1. Preheat oven to 325°. Apply cooking spray to the 12-cup muffin tin. Put a large skillet over medium heat and heat the oil. Cook the onions and potatoes. Season with ¼ teaspoon of salt. Keep stirring while you cook for about 5 minutes or until the potatoes are cooked through. Remove the skillet from the heat.

2. In a large bowl, whisk the eggs, milk, cheese, remaining salt, and pepper. Add the spinach and the potato mixture.

3. Pour the mixture into the muffin cups and bake for about 25 minutes or until the quiche is firm to the touch. After cooking, let it stand for about 5 minutes before removing from the tin.

4. Wrap each in quiche in a plastic bag. Refrigerate (for up to 3 days) or freeze (for up to 1 month).

5. Remove the quiches from their plastic bags and wrap each in a paper towel before reheating. Microwave them on high for 30-60 seconds.

Avocado-Egg Sandwich

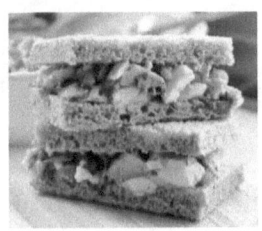

Servings: 5
Nutritional Information: Calories- 350; Fats- 19g; Carbohydrates- 30g; Protein- 17g

Ingredients

- 1½ ripe avocado
- 6 hard-boiled eggs, chopped
- ¼ cup celery, finely chopped
- 2 tbsp. fresh chives, snipped
- 2 tsp. lemon juice
- 2 tsp. avocado oil
- ¼ tsp. salt
- ¼ tsp. ground pepper
- 10 slices whole-wheat sandwich bread, toasted
- 5 lettuce leaves

Directions

1. Using a spoon, scoop out the avocado flesh into a medium bowl. Add the oil and lemon juice before mashing the flesh. The consistency for this doesn't need to be smooth. There should be bits of chunks left for the texture.

2. Add the chives, celery, and chopped eggs. Season with salt and pepper and mix well. Divide the mixture between 5 bread slices, put lettuce on top, and cover with the remaining slices.

Lemony Linguine with Spring Vegetables

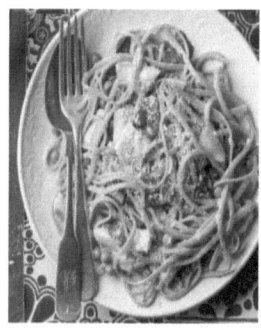

Servings: 5
Nutritional Information: Calories- 372; Fats- 7g; Carbohydrates- 64g; Protein- 18g

Ingredients

- 8 oz. whole-wheat linguine
- 1 x 9 oz. package frozen artichoke hearts
- 6 cups mature spinach, chopped
- 2 cups peas, fresh or frozen
- ¼ cup Parmesan cheese (plus ¼ cup for serving), freshly grated
- ¼ cup half-and-half
- 4 cloves garlic, thinly sliced
- 3½ cups water
- 1 tbsp. lemon zest
- 3-4 tbsp. lemon juice
- ¼ tsp. ground pepper
- ½ tsp. salt

Directions

1. In a large pot, combine the pasta, garlic, pepper, and salt. Place over high heat and bring to a boil. Continue to boil for about 8 minutes, stirring frequently.

2. Add the spinach, artichokes, and peas then stir. Continue to cook for about 2-4 minutes or until the pasta is tender and most of the liquid has evaporated.

3. Remove the pan from heat and sprinkle ¼ cup of freshly grated parmesan, half-and-half, lemon juice, and lemon zest. Let it stand for 5 minutes, stirring occasionally.

4. To serve, sprinkle with ¼ cup of freshly grated parmesan.

Banana Bran Muffins

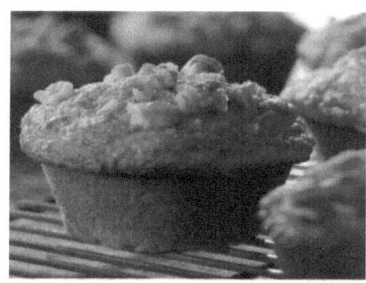

Servings: 12
Nutritional Information: Calories- 200; Fats- 6g; Carbohydrates- 34g; Protein- 5g

Ingredients

- 1 cup ripe bananas, mashed
- 1 cup unprocessed wheat bran
- 1 cup whole-wheat flour
- 1 cup buttermilk
- ¾ cup all-purpose flour
- ⅔ cup packed light brown sugar
- ¼ cup canola oil
- 1½ tsp. baking powder
- 2 large eggs
- 1 tsp. vanilla extract
- ½ tsp. baking soda
- ½ tsp. ground cinnamon
- ¼ tsp. salt
- ½ cup chocolate chips
- ⅓ cup chopped walnuts

Directions

1. Preheat oven to 400°. Apply cooking spray on muffin cups.

2. In a medium bowl, whisk the sugar and eggs together. Whisk in the bananas, vanilla, bran, buttermilk, and oil.

3. With the exception of chocolate chips and walnuts, mix all the remaining dry ingredients in a large mixing bowl. Create a well at the center and throw in all wet mixtures into it.

4. Add the batter to the muffin cups and sprinkle with walnuts.

5. Bake for 15-25 minutes or until the tops are golden. You can also perform the toothpick test to know if they're ready. Let them cool before transferring them to your storage container.

Tuscan Bean and Kale Stew

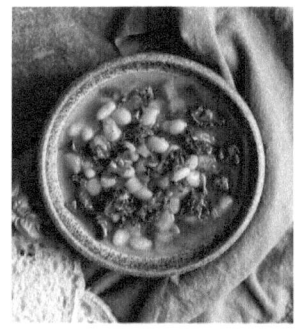

Servings: 5
Nutritional Information: Calories- 307; Fats- 11g; Carbohydrates- 28.5g; Protein- 26g

Ingredients

- 12 oz. raw, mild Italian turkey sausage, cut into 1-inch chunks
- 2 cups BPA-free canned cannellini beans
- 2 cups baby spinach
- 2 cups kale, shredded
- 3 cups grape tomatoes
- 2 cups low-sodium chicken broth
- 2 pinches saffron threads
- ½ tsp. dried thyme
- 2 small shallots, thinly sliced
- 2 cloves garlic, minced
- 2 tsp. olive oil
- ¼ tsp. ground black pepper
- 1/8 tsp. sea salt

Directions

1. Place a small saucepan over medium heat and bring the broth to a simmer. Add the saffron threads, remove the pan from the heat, and set aside.

2. Put a large saucepan over medium-high heat and pour oil. Brown the sausage for about 5-7 minutes.

3. Add the garlic, shallots, and thyme. Season with salt and pepper. Stir for about 2 minutes or until the garlic and shallots are fragrant.

4. Add the beans, tomatoes, and the chicken broth. Bring the mixture to a simmer and reduce the heat to medium-low. Let it simmer for about 15 minutes.

5. Place the spinach and kale. Stir occasionally and let it cook for another 1-2 minutes or until the leaves have wilted.

Burmese Chicken

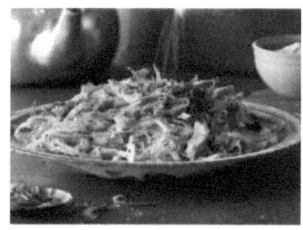

Servings: 5
Nutritional Information: Calories- 335; Fats- 22g; Carbohydrates- 10g; Protein- 23g

Ingredients

- 1 lb. boneless and skinless chicken thighs
- 3 cups cabbage, shredded
- ½ cup fresh cilantro, coarsely chopped
- ⅓ cup shallots, halved and sliced
- 3 tbsp. lime juice
- ¼ cup canola oil
- ¼ tsp. red pepper, crushed
- 1½ tbsp. chickpea flour, toasted and divided
- 2 tsp. fish sauce
- ⅓ cup fried shallots, for garnish

Directions

1. Put the chicken thighs in a large saucepan and cover them with water. Bring the water to a boil.

2. Reduce the heat to a simmer as soon as it boils. Cover the pan with a lid and cook for 6-8 minutes. (You can also use an instant-read thermometer to know if the chicken is cooked. Insert it in the thickest part of the thigh and if the temperature reads 165°F, then it's done.)

3. Once done, transfer the chicken thighs on a clean cutting board and let it rest for about 5 minutes. When the chicken is already cool to your touch, shred it.

4. Meanwhile, mix the lime juice and shallots in a serving bowl. Set it aside for 5 minutes. After that, whisk the fish sauce, red pepper, and oil together with the shallots.

5. Add the chicken, a tablespoon of chickpea flour, cabbage, and cilantro. Mix them all together until well combined. To serve, garnish the salad with the remaining flour and fried shallots.

Squash and Red Lentil Curry

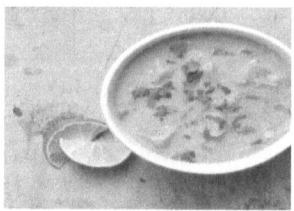

Servings: 5
Nutritional Information: Calories- 326; Fats- 12g; Carbohydrates- 46g; Protein- 14g

Ingredients

- 1 cup red lentils
- 1 x 20oz. package cubed and peeled butternut squash
- 1 x 14oz. can lite coconut milk
- 2 cloves garlic, minced
- 1½ cups onion, diced
- 1 tbsp. fresh ginger, minced
- 4 cups water
- 1 cup fresh tomato, chopped
- 2 tsp. garam masala or curry powder
- 2 tbsp. canola oil
- 1½ tsp. salt
- 5 lime wedges, for serving
- Fresh cilantro, chopped for garnish

Directions

1. Heat oil in a large pot placed over medium-high heat. Sauté the onions, ginger, and garlic. Add the garam masala (or curry powder) and cook for about 2-3 minutes or until the onions have softened. Remember to stir often.

2. Add the lentils, squash, and tomatoes. Season with salt. Cook for another 1 minute. Add water and cover the pot with a lid.

Bring it to a boil. Once it boils, immediately reduce heat and let it simmer.

3. Stir occasionally and cook until the squash is tender, and the lentils have crumbled. This should take about 20 minutes.

4. Stir in the coconut milk and let it maintain a gentle simmer for about a minute.

5. To serve, top with chopped cilantro and lime wedges on the side.

Poached Cod and Green Lentil Beans with Pesto

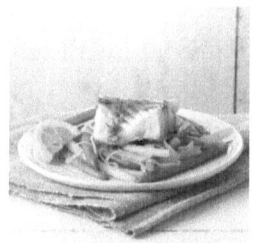

Servings: 5-6
Nutritional Information: Calories- 264; Fats- 12g; Carbohydrates- 15g; Protein- 26g

Ingredients

- 1¼ - 2 lb. cod
- 1 lb. green and/or yellow wax beans, trimmed
- 1½ cups low-sodium chicken broth
- ¾ cup shallot, thinly sliced
- ¼ cup homemade pesto
- 1 tbsp. extra-virgin olive oil
- ¼ tsp. salt
- ¼ tsp. freshly ground pepper
- Lemon wedges, for serving

Directions

1. Place a large skillet over medium-high heat and heat the oil. Add the shallots and beans, stirring occasionally. Cook for about 1-2 minutes or until the shallots soften.

2. Season both sides of the cod with salt and pepper. Spread the beans in the bottom of the pan and put the cod on top.

3. Raise the heat to high and add the broth. Cover the pan with a lid and continue to cook for 4-6 minutes or until the cod is

cooked through. Using a slotted spoon, move the cod and beans to a container.

4. Meanwhile, cook the broth over high heat for about 5 minutes. Do not cover the pan so it will be reduced to half a cup. Remove from the heat and add the pesto. Let the sauce cool before storing.

5. To serve, pour the sauce over the cod and beans. Put lemon wedges on the side.

Mexican Chicken Avocado Salad

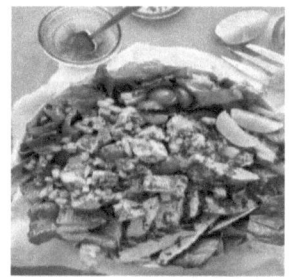

Servings: 5
Nutritional Information: Calories- 277; Fats- 16.3g; Carbohydrates- 9.8g; Protein- 23.5g

Ingredients

- 2 boneless and skinless chicken breasts, fresh or frozen
- 1 avocado, diced
- 1 red bell pepper, diced
- 1/3 red onion, diced
- 1 jalapeño, diced
- 1/8 cup cilantro, finely chopped
- ¼ cup plain Greek yogurt
- 2 tbsp. homemade ranch dressing
- 1 tbsp. lime juice
- 1 ½ tsp. garlic powder
- 1 tsp. pepper
- ½ tsp. chili powder
- ½ tsp. salt

Directions

1. Pour water into the pot and add the salt. Bring it to a boil and add the chicken. Cook it for 20 minutes (for fresh) and 40 minutes (for frozen) or until the chicken is cooked through.

2. Meanwhile, put the vegetables and herbs in a bowl. In a separate bowl, combine the avocado, ranch dressing, yogurt, spices, and lime juice together.

3. Dice or shred (according to your preference) the chicken once it was done. Mix everything together before storing in a container (or containers). Refrigerate.

Parsley & Garlic Chicken Cutlets with Broccoli

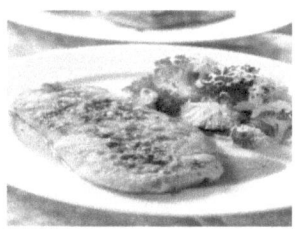

Servings: 5
Nutritional Information: Calories- 486; Fats- 19g; Carbohydrates- 15.7g; Protein- 54g

Ingredients

- 8-10 organic chicken cutlets
- 16 oz. fresh organic broccoli florets
- 1/3 cup whole wheat pastry flour
- 3/4 cup dry white wine
- 4 garlic cloves, chopped
- 2 tbsp. butter, cut into pieces
- 4 tbsp. fresh parsley, chopped
- 3 tbsp. olive oil, divided
- ¼ tsp. Celtic sea salt

Directions

1. Pour flour on a large plate and proceed to coat the chicken. Place a large, non-stick skillet over medium-high heat and heat half of the oil. Cook the chicken in batches, with each side cooked in 3-5 minutes.

2. Meanwhile, microwave the broccoli for about 5-7 minutes.

3. When the all the chicken cutlets are cooked, transfer them to a container and set aside.

4. Using the same skillet where you fried the chicken, add the garlic and cook until it's fragrant. Add the wine and reduce it by half. This may take about 3 minutes.

5. Once the wine has been reduced, turn off the heat. Add the butter, salt, and parsley. Pour the mixture of the chicken and add the broccoli. Store.

Low-Carb Mexican Casserole

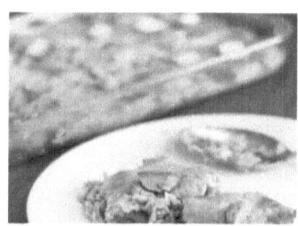

Servings: 12
Nutritional Information: Calories- 69.42; Fats- 11g; Carbohydrates- 2.83g; Protein- 4.56g

Ingredients

- 8 cherry tomatoes, halved
- 1 head cauliflower
- 1½ cups cheese, divided
- 1 green bell pepper, diced
- 1 red bell pepper, diced
- ½ white onion
- 1 jalapeno, diced
- 1 tsp. chili powder
- 1 tsp. cumin

Directions

1. Preheat oven to 350° F. Meanwhile, warm a skillet over medium heat. Cook the peppers, onions, chili powder, and cumin. Stir every 2 minutes. Make sure to properly roast the peppers. Once done remove the skillet from the heat and set aside.

2. Using a box grater or food processor, rice the cauliflower and microwave it for 3 minutes. In a large bowl, mix the tomatoes, 1 cup of cheese, riced cauliflower, and the roasted pepper mixture.

3. Coat a 7x11.6x2" baking dish with cooking spray. Pour and spread the casserole mixture into the baking dish. Top it with the remaining cheese. Bake it for about 30-35 minutes or until the cheese is melted.

Spiced Tempeh Tacos with Creamy Cashew Sauce

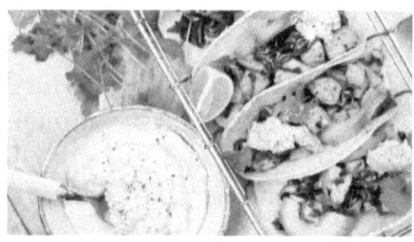

Servings: 5
Nutritional Information: Calories- 341; Fats- 20g; Carbohydrates- 29g; Protein- 4g

Ingredients

For the cashew sauce:

- ½ cup raw unsalted cashews
- 1/3 cup fresh lime juice
- 1 ½ tsp. ancho chili powder
- ½ tsp. garlic powder
- 5 tbsp. water
- A pinch of sea salt
- A pinch of black pepper

For the tacos:

- 8 x 5-inch corn tortillas, warmed
- 1 x 8 oz. package organic tempeh, cubed
- 1 yellow onion, thinly sliced
- 1 tsp. chili powder
- ½ tsp. ground cumin
- 2 tbsp. coconut oil
- ½ tsp. sea salt
- 1/8 tsp. ground black pepper

Directions

1. To prepare the sauce, process all the sauce ingredients in a blender or food processor until smooth.

2. For the tacos, put a large skillet over medium-high heat and heat the oil. Cook the onions for 3-4 minutes. Add cumin, chili powder, salt, and pepper and stir for 30 seconds. Put the tempeh and cook for another 3-4 minutes.

3. To arrange, divide the tempeh mixture among the tortillas. To serve, top with cashew sauce and other garnishes (*see meal plan*).

Crispy Fried Salmon with Spring Vegetable Broth

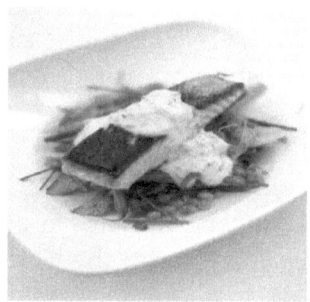

Servings: 5
Nutritional Information: Calories- 337; Fats- 19.5g; Carbohydrates- 8g; Protein- 29.7g

Ingredients

- 5 x 120g salmon steaks, scored
- 850 ml organic chicken or vegetable stock, lightly seasoned
- 8 baby bulbs fennel, stalks removed
- 100g green beans, tops removed
- 100g podded peas
- 100g podded broad beans
- A handful fresh basil, leaves picked and ripped
- A handful fresh mint, ripped
- Extra virgin olive oil
- Sea salt
- Freshly ground black pepper
- Aioli

Directions

1. In a large saucepan over medium-high heat, bring the stock to a boil. Add the fennel and continue to boil for 4 minutes.

2. While you're at it, heat a non-stick for the salmon. Before placing the fish, to the pan, you can finely slice a bit your basil and mint and push them into the score marks.

3. Brush the steaks with olive oil and season with salt and pepper. Put the salmon with the skin-side down and cook for 2 minutes on each side.

4. After 4 minutes on the broth, add the broad beans and green beans. Cook for another 2 minutes and add the peas. Cook for another 2 minutes and turn off the heat.

5. Divide the broth among containers and add the ripped basil and mint. Place the salmon on top. To serve, add a dollop of aioli.

Fish Sticks

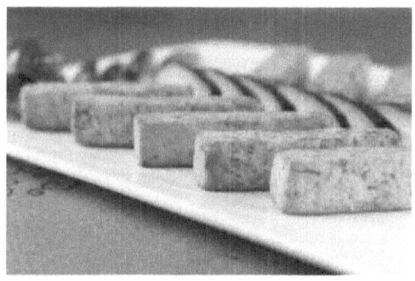

Servings: 5
Nutritional Information: Calories- 303; Fats- 4g; Carbohydrates- 37g; Protein- 31g

Ingredients

- 1 lb. tilapia fillets, cut into ½x3" strips
- 1 cup whole-grain cereal flakes
- 1 cup whole-wheat dry breadcrumbs
- 1 tsp. lemon pepper
- ½ tsp. garlic powder
- ½ tsp. paprika
- 2 large egg whites, beaten
- ½ cup all-purpose flour
- Canola oil cooking spray
- ¼ tsp. salt

Directions

1. Preheat oven to 450°F. Put a wire rack on a baking sheet and coat them with cooking spray. Set aside. Using a food processor or blender, process the cereal flakes, bread crumbs, garlic powder, lemon pepper, paprika, and salt until finely ground. Transfer the mixture to a plate.

2. Put flour on another plate and the egg whites on a third one. Coat each fish strip with flour one at a time; next, dip in the egg white; and lastly into the breadcrumb mixture.

3. Arrange the strips on the rack and coat both sides with cooking spray. Bake for 10 minutes or until they're golden brown.

Salisbury Steak with Mushroom Gravy

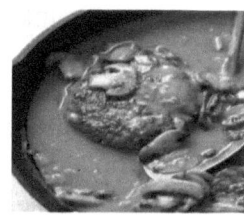

Servings: 5
Nutritional Information: Calories- 262; Fats- 13.5g; Carbohydrates- 8g; Protein- 1.5g

Ingredients

- 1 lb. lean ground beef
- 1 cup low-sodium beef broth
- 4 oz. wild mushrooms, trimmed and sliced
- 1 tbsp. fresh thyme leaves
- 1 tbsp. unsalted tomato paste
- 1 clove garlic, minced
- 1 small red onion, thinly sliced
- 2 tsp. organic unsalted butter
- 1½ tbsp. white whole-wheat flour
- 2 tsp. Dijon mustard
- 2 tbsp. Worcestershire sauce, divided
- 1 tsp. balsamic vinegar
- 1 tbsp. safflower oil, divided
- 3/4 tsp. ground black pepper, divided
- 3/4 tsp. sea salt, divided

Direction

1. In a large bowl, incorporate the beef, tomato paste, mustard, thyme, 1½ tbsp. Worcestershire sauce and a half teaspoon each of salt and pepper. Form five patties and sprinkle each side with remaining salt and pepper.

2. Place a large skillet over medium-high heat and heat oil. Fry the patties for 8-10 minutes, turning it from time-to-time. See to it that the inside is no longer pink. Transfer to a plate.

3. Reduce heat to medium and melt the butter. Cook the onion, stirring occasionally for about 4 minutes or until it's softened. Add the mushrooms and cook, stirring frequently for about 3-4 minutes.

4. Sprinkle flour on mushroom mixture and stir continually for about a minute.

5. Add the broth, remaining Worcestershire sauce, and vinegar. Bring to a simmer and reduce heat to low. Continue to simmer for about 4-5 minutes or at least until the gravy thickens. To serve, top the patties with the gravy.

Southwestern Turkey Quinoa Stuffed Peppers

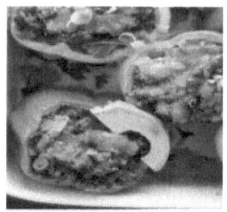

Servings: 7
Nutritional Information: Calories- 262; Fats- 9g; Carbohydrates- 22g; Protein- 23g

Ingredients

- 7 large bell peppers (assorted colors), tops cut off and seeds removed
- 1 lb. ground lean turkey
- 15 oz. Muir Glen fire-roasted tomatoes, diced
- 1 large chipotle pepper, minced
- ¾ cup frozen corn
- ¾ cup black beans, drained and rinsed
- ¾ cup Colby jack cheese, shredded
- ½ cup dried quinoa
- ¼ cup fresh cilantro, diced
- 1 red onion, diced
- 3 garlic cloves
- 2 tbsp. olive oil
- 1 tsp. cumin
- 1 tsp. smoked paprika
- ¼ tsp. ground black pepper
- ½ tsp. salt

Directions

1. Preheat oven to 350°. Add a cup of water in a small saucepan. Place over medium-high heat and bring to a boil. Add the

quinoa and cover with lid. Bring again to a boil and then reduce heat. Simmer for about 10-13 minutes or until the water has evaporated. Fluff the quinoa with a fork and set aside to cool.

2. Place a large skillet over medium-high heat and heat olive oil. Cook the onions for 2-3 minutes or until translucent. Add the chipotle peppers and garlic and sauté for another minute. Add the turkey and cook for 5-7 minutes or until no longer pinkish.

3. Add the black beans, corn, tomatoes, tomatoes, paprika, cumin, and cilantro. Season with salt. Cook for 4-5 minutes or until the liquid has evaporated. Stir occasionally.

4. Transfer the quinoa and turkey mixture to a bowl and toss. Arrange the bell peppers in 13x9" baking dish with the open-side up. Stuff each with the quinoa-turkey mixture and bake for 40 minutes.

5. Remove from the oven and top each stuffed pepper with 1 tbsp. of freshly grated cheese. Put back into the oven and cook for another minute or until the cheese is melted. To serve, you can top each stuffed pepper with sliced green onions, diced cilantro, and avocado slices.

Swedish Meatballs

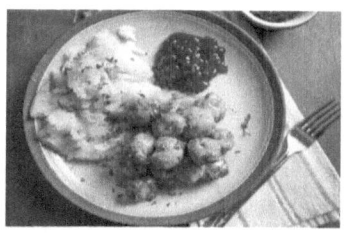

Servings: 5
Nutritional Information: Calories- 213.5; Fats- 10g; Carbohydrates- 8.5g; Protein- 25.1g

Ingredients

- 1 lb. 93% lean ground beef
- 2 oz. light cream cheese
- ¼ cup seasoned breadcrumbs
- 1 large egg
- 1 celery stalk, minced
- 1 small onion, minced
- 1 clove garlic, minced
- ¼ cup minced parsley
- ½ tsp. allspice
- 1 tsp. olive oil
- 2 cups reduced sodium beef stock
- Salt
- Pepper

Directions

1. Heat oil in a large skillet over medium heat. Sauté onions and garlic for about 4-5 minutes or until the onions are translucent. Add the parsley and celery and cook for another 3-4 minutes. Turn off heat and let it cool for a couple of minutes.

2. After the cooling period, make the meatballs. In a large mixing bowl, add the beef, breadcrumbs, allspice, and onion mixture. Season with salt and pepper. Combine the ingredients well and form the balls. Use 1/8 cup of the mixture to form one ball.

3. When you're finished forming the balls, add the beef stock to the pan where you cooked the onions and bring it to a boil. Reduce the heat to medium-low after boiling and drop the balls to the stock. For your safety, use a ladle or slotted spoon to drop the balls. Cover the skillet with a lid and cook for about 20 minutes.

4. Remove the meatballs using a slotted spoon and set it aside. Strain the stock and transfer it to a blender together with cream cheese. Process until smooth.

5. Transfer the mixture to the pan and simmer for a few minutes in order to achieve a thick consistency. Place both the meatballs and the sauce in your storage container and freeze.

Shrimp Ceviche and Avocado Salad

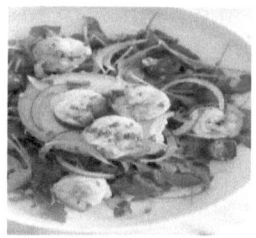

Servings: 5
Nutritional Information: Calories- 254; Fats- 16g; Carbohydrates- 13g; Protein- 18g

Ingredients

- 11 oz. extra-large shrimp, cleaned and deveined
- 12 grape or cherry tomatoes, halved
- 2 tbsp. cilantro, finely chopped
- 1/8 tsp cumin
- ½ red onion, sliced
- ½ jalapeno, finely diced
- 2 garlic cloves, crushed
- ¼ cup white wine vinegar
- 2 tbsp. clam juice
- 1 tsp kosher salt
- 1 tbsp. olive oil
- 1/8 tsp pepper
- ½ tsp. raw honey
- Haas avocados, to serve
- Arugula, to serve

Directions

1. To blanch the shrimp, bring a large pot of water to a boil. Add the shrimp and cook for about 4 minutes or until opaque. Remove from the pot and submerge them in an ice bath.

2. In a large mixing bowl, incorporate the tomatoes, onions, jalapeno, garlic, cilantro, clam juice, cumin, honey, olive oil, wine vinegar, salt, and pepper. Add the shrimp, divide among storage containers and refrigerate.

3. To serve, put the flesh of half avocado and arugula leaves on plate and top with ceviche.

Cauliflower Risotto with Seared Scallops

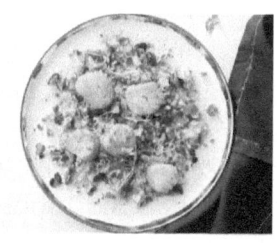

Servings: 5-6
Nutritional Information: Calories- 262; Fats- 11g; Carbohydrates- 21g; Protein- 23g

Ingredients

- 7 cups cauliflower florets (about 1 head)
- 1 lb. sea scallops, patted dry
- 2 cups asparagus, trimmed and cut into 1-inch pieces
- 3/4 cup low-sodium chicken broth
- ½ cup Parmesan cheese, freshly grated
- 3 tbsp. whole milk
- 1 tbsp. organic unsalted butter, cut into small pieces and chilled
- 1 tbsp. lemon zest
- 2 tbsp. fresh chives, chopped
- 2 cloves garlic, minced
- 2 tbsp. unsalted pine nuts
- 1 tbsp. olive oil, divided
- 1 tsp. ground black pepper, divided
- ½ tsp. sea salt, divided

Directions

1. For this step, you can work in batches. Rice the cauliflower florets in a food processor and set aside. Place a 12-inch skillet over medium-high heat and heat 1½ tsp. oil. Using silicone

brush, spread the oil all over the pan. Cook the garlic, stirring often, for about 30 seconds or until fragrant.

2. Add the riced cauliflower and season with ½ tsp. pepper and ¼ tsp. salt. Cook, stirring occasionally, for 4-5 minutes or until the cauliflower is golden. Add the broth and cook for another 2 minutes. Remove about 1 cup of the broth mixture and transfer it to the food processor. Add milk and grated parmesan and process until smooth.

3. Add back to the skillet and stir well. Add the asparagus and cover the pan with a lid. Continue to cook for 3-4 minutes or until the asparagus is tender. Stir in butter before transferring to a bowl. Add pine nuts, 1 ½ tbsp. chives, and lemon zest. Cover the bowl. Wipe skillet with paper towel and add the remaining oil. Set heat to medium-high and spread oil using silicone brush.

4. Season scallops with remaining salt and pepper. Cook them for about 2-3 minutes or until the bottoms are browned. To check if they're done, try to lift them using a spatula. If they still stick to the pan, cook for another 30 seconds. Flip and cook for another 1 ½- 2 minutes or until the bottoms are browned. The scallops should be slightly firm but soft when pressed.

5. Divide risotto among containers and top with scallops. Drizzle with sauce and garnish with chives. Store in freezer.

Mac & Cheese with Collards

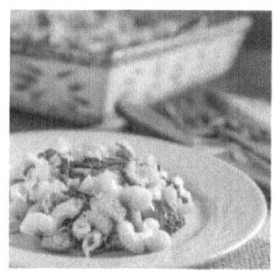

Servings: 5
Nutritional Information: Calories-470; Fats- 19g; Carbohydrates- 57g; Protein- 22g

Ingredients

- 2 cups whole-wheat elbow noodles
- 1 cup extra-sharp Cheddar cheese, shredded
- 4 cups collard greens, chopped
- 2 oz. reduced-fat cream cheese
- 1¾ cups low-fat milk, divided
- ¼ cup panko breadcrumbs, preferably whole-wheat
- 3 tbsp. all-purpose flour
- 2 tsp. white-wine vinegar
- ½ tsp. paprika
- 1 tbsp. extra-virgin olive oil
- ¼ tsp. ground pepper
- ½ tsp. salt

Directions

1. Place a large pot of water over medium-high heat and bring it to a boil. Add the pasta and collards and cook according to the pasta package instructions. Drain. Place a large broiler-safe skillet over medium-high heat and heat 1 ½ cups of milk until it simmers.

2. In a small bowl, mix the remaining milk, flour, pepper, and salt. Add this mixture to the simmering milk and reduce the heat to medium-low. Continue to cook for about a minute or two, whisking constantly until it thickens.

3. Remove the pan from the heat and add the cream cheese, cheddar, and vinegar. Whisk until the cheese is melted. Add the pasta and collards to the sauce. Place the rack in upper third of the oven and preheat the broiler to high.

4. In a small bowl, mix the breadcrumbs, paprika, and oil together. Sprinkle this over the pasta. Broil the pasta for about 1-3 minutes or until golden brown. Cool completely before freezing.

Mini Pepperoni Pizza

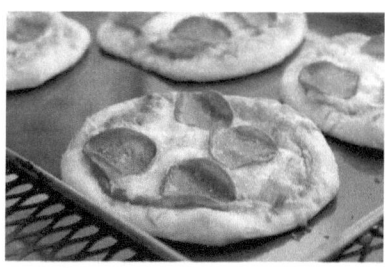

Servings: 5
Nutritional Information: Calories-138; Fats- 7g; Carbohydrates- 13g; Protein- 6g

Ingredients

- 5 tbsp. mini pepperoni
- 5 - 1x 6-inch corn tortilla
- 10 tbsp. part-skim mozzarella cheese, shredded
- 1/3 pizza sauce

Directions

1. Preheat oven to 400°. Spread pizza sauce onto the tortilla. Sprinkle mozzarella on top and assemble the pepperoni on top of this.

2. Place on 5 small baking sheets and bake for 6-8 minutes or until the cheese is bubbling and the tortilla has crisped.

Steak Skewers with Strawberry Chimichurri

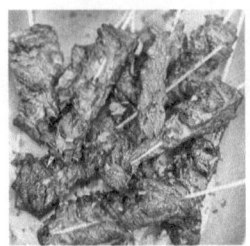

Servings: 10
Nutritional Information: Calories- 272; Fats- 17g; Carbohydrates- 5g; Protein- 25g

Ingredients

- 1 lb. skirt steak, trimmed
- 3/4 cup strawberries, finely diced
- 3/4 cup parsley, chopped
- ¼ cup extra-virgin olive oil
- 3 tsp. oregano, chopped
- 1 tsp. thyme, chopped
- 1 small shallot, minced
- ¼ tsp. cayenne pepper
- 2 tsp. cumin
- 1 tbsp. chili powder
- 2 tsp. honey
- 2 tbsp. red wine vinegar
- 3/4 tsp. black pepper
- 3/4 tsp. kosher salt

Directions

1. First, soak 10 wooden skewers in water for about half an hour. Meanwhile, mix the strawberries, parsley, oregano, thyme, shallot, olive oil, wine vinegar, honey, ½ tsp. each of salt and pepper in a medium mixing bowl.

2. Try to cut the steak into 10 equal-sized strips about 1-inch wide. Place them in a large bowl. Add the cayenne, cumin, and chili powders. Season with the remaining salt and pepper. Mix well to coat. When the skewers are ready, thread the steak strips into them.

3. Coat the grill with cooking spray and adjust heat to very high. Arrange the skewers on the grill and cook for 2-3 minutes on each side (for medium-rare) or more for your desired doneness. Transfer to a clean cutting board to cool completely.

Freezer Beans and Cheese Burritos

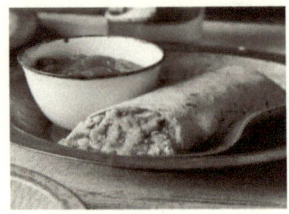

Servings: 8
Nutritional Information: Calories- 336; Fats- 12g; Carbohydrates- 41g; Protein- 15g

Ingredients

- 8 x 8-inch whole-wheat tortillas
- 1½ cups chopped grape tomatoes
- 2 cups sharp Cheddar cheese, shredded
- 2 x 15oz. can low-sodium pinto beans, rinsed
- 4 scallions, chopped
- ¼ cup pickled jalapeño peppers, chopped
- 2 tbsp. fresh cilantro, chopped
- 4 tsp. chili powder
- 1 tsp. ground cumin

Directions

1. In a medium bowl, mix the tomatoes, cilantro, jalapeños, and scallions together. In a large bowl, mash the beans together with cumin and chili powder using a potato masher or fork until almost smooth.

2. Add the tomato mixture and cheese and stir until combined. Spread about half a cup of the filling mixture on the bottom third of each tortilla. Roll the tortillas securely, tucking in the ends as you go. Wrap each roll with a sturdy aluminum foil and freeze.

3. To heat, unwrap the burrito and put in a microwave-safe plate or dish. Cover them with a paper towel (or towels) and microwave on high for about 1 ½- 2 ½ minutes.

Spaghetti with Quick Meat Sauce

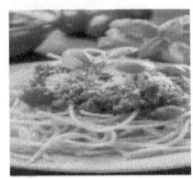

Servings: 8
Nutritional Information: Calories- 389; Fats- 9g; Carbohydrates- 54g; Protein- 27g

Ingredients

- 1 lb. whole-wheat spaghetti
- 1 lb. lean (90% or leaner) ground beef
- ½ cup Parmesan cheese, freshly grated
- 1 x 28oz. can crushed tomatoes
- 1 large carrot, finely chopped
- 1 stalk celery, finely chopped
- 1 large onion, finely chopped
- 4 cloves garlic, minced
- 1 tbsp. Italian seasoning
- ¼ cup flat-leaf parsley, chopped
- 2 tsp. extra-virgin olive oil
- ½ tsp. salt

Directions

1. Put a large pot of water over medium-high heat and bring to a boil. Cook the pasta according to package instructions. Drain.

2. Meanwhile, place skillet over medium heat and heat the oil. Add the carrots, celery, and onions. Cook for about 5-8 minutes or until the onions begin to brown. Add the garlic and Italian seasoning and stir well. Cook for another 30 seconds or until fragrant.

3. Add the beef and use a spoon to break it. Cook for 3-5 minutes or until the meat is no longer pink. Adjust the heat to high and stir in the tomatoes.

4. Cook for about 4-6 minutes or until the mixture has thickened. Add parsley and salt.

5. Refrigerate the pasta and sauce for up to three days or freeze for up to a month. To serve, sprinkle with cheese.

Peanut Butter-Oat Energy Balls

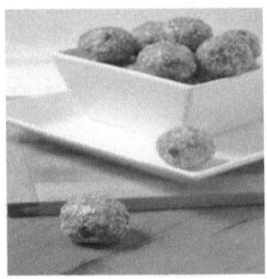

Servings: 12
Nutritional Information: Calories- 73; Fats- 3g; Carbohydrates- 10g; Protein- 2g

Ingredients

- ¾ cup Medjool dates, chopped
- ½ cup rolled oats
- ¼ cup natural peanut butter
- Chia seeds, for garnish

Directions

1. In a small bowl, soak the dates in hot water for 5-10 minutes. Drain.

2. In a food processor, process the oats, peanut butter, and soaked dates until very finely chopped. Roll them into 12 balls and garnish with chia seeds.

3. Store in an airtight container and refrigerate for up to a week.

Mango Fruit Leather

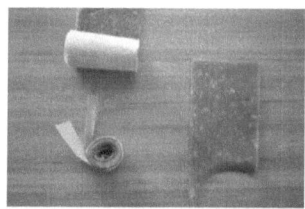

Servings: 7
Nutritional Information (1 fruit leather): Calories- 87; Fats- 1g; Carbohydrates- 22g; Protein- 1g

Ingredients

- 3 large ripe mangoes, peeled
- 1 tsp. lemon juice
- ½ cup water

Directions

1. Preheat oven to 200°. Prepare a large rimmed baking sheet by lining it with a non-stick baking mat.

2. Cut the mango flesh away from the pit and transfer directly to a blender. Add the lemon juice and water. Process until smooth.

3. Pour the puree into a medium saucepan over medium heat. Bring it to a simmer and reduce heat. Maintain a gentle simmer and continue to cook for another 20 minutes or until it is reduced to 2 cups.

4. Pour the puree on the baking sheet and spread it evenly using a rubber spatula. Form a thin rectangle, about 1/8-inch thick and bake for 4-6 hours or until it's dry to the touch. Let it cool completely.

5. Transfer the fruit leather to a wax paper or parchment paper of the same size. Leave the paper underneath as you roll the fruit leather into a long cylinder.

6. Using a pair of scissors or a sharp knife, cut the mango fruit leather into 2-inch wide strips. Store this in an airtight container for up to 1 week.

Peanut Butter Banana Cups

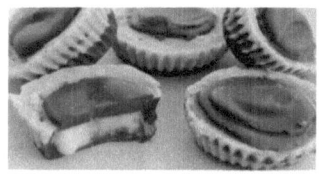

Servings: 16
Nutritional Information: Calories- 69; Fats- 4g; Carbohydrates- 11g; Protein- 1g

Ingredients

- 3/4 cup chocolate chips
- 1 medium banana, peeled and divided into 16 rounds
- ¼ cup all-natural homemade peanut butter
- 1 tbsp. unrefined coconut oil, melted

Directions

1. Line the countertop with wax sheets or parchment paper then arrange 16 pieces of 1.25-inch baking cups on top. Melt the chocolate chips using a double-boiler and allow to cool it slightly. Meanwhile, incorporate the peanut butter and coconut oil.

2. Pour about a teaspoon of melted chocolate at the bottom of each cup. Next, set a banana slice on top, then a teaspoon of peanut butter. Lastly, drop about half a teaspoon of chocolate at the middle of each cup.

3. Transfer the cups to a casserole pan or a freezer-safe dish and place it on a freezer. The peanut butter banana cups will be ready in an hour. To thaw, just set the cups at room temperature for 2-3 minutes.

Apple Nachos

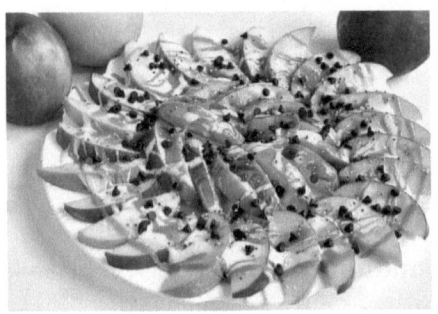

Servings: 5
Nutritional Information: Calories- 231; Fats- 13g; Carbohydrates- 31g; Protein- 3g

Ingredients

- 3 tart apples, cored, peeled and cut into ¼" cubes
- 2 tsp. lemon juice
- ½ cup dark chocolate chips
- ¼ cup diced pecans
- ½ cup caramel sauce

Directions

1. Combine the apples, lemon juice, and chocolate chips in a large mixing bowl. Refrigerate. To serve, drizzle with hot caramel sauce.

Fried Shallots

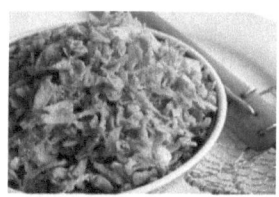

Servings: 1 cup
Nutritional Information (per teaspoon): Calories- 10; Fats- 1g; Carbohydrates- 0g; Protein- 0g

Ingredient

- ½ cup shallots, halved and sliced

Directions

1. Put a fine-mesh strainer over a heatproof bowl. Place a small skillet over medium-high heat and heat half cup canola oil. Put the shallots into the pan and reduce heat into a medium. Cook the shallots for about 3-5 minutes or until golden brown.

2. Pour the shallots and oil through the strainer. Transfer the shallots to a plate lined with paper towels. Set aside until completely cooled. As for the oil, you can reserve it if you want to.

3. When the shallots are already cool, transfer them to an airtight container and store it at room temperature for up to 7 days. You can refrigerate the oil for 2 months.

Homemade Pesto Sauce

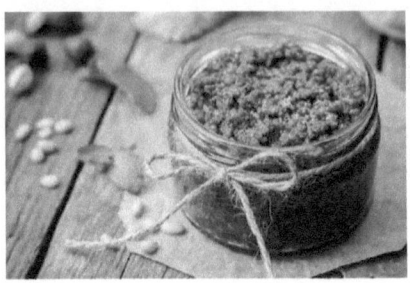

Servings: 2 ¼ cups
Nutritional Information (per tablespoon): Calories- 80; Fats- 7.51g; Carbohydrates- 0.76g; Protein- 2.71g

Ingredients

- 1 cup fresh basil
- 7 medium cloves garlic
- ½ cup roasted pine nuts
- ½ cup olive oil
- 1 cup parmesan cheese
- Salt to taste

Directions

1. Put all the ingredients in a blender or food processor. Process until you achieve a smooth pesto sauce.

Clean Eating Ranch Dressing

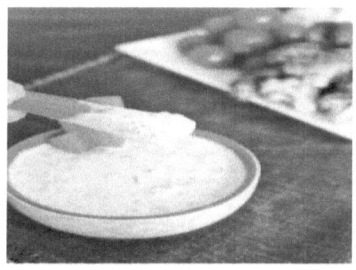

Servings: 1 cup
Nutritional Information (per tablespoon): Calories- 11; Fats- 7.51g; Carbohydrates- 1g; Protein- 1g

Ingredients

- 3 tbsp. plain Greek yogurt
- 5 tbsp. buttermilk
- ¼ tsp. dried dill
- ¼ tsp. onion powder
- ½ tsp. dried chives
- ½ tsp. dried parsley
- ½ tsp. salt
- ground black pepper

Directions

1. Using a spoon or whisk, combine all the ingredients together in a bowl until a smooth consistency is achieved.

Aioli

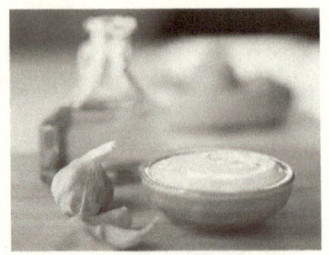

Servings: 8
Nutritional Information: Calories- 498; Fats- 54.9g; Carbohydrates- 0.4g; Protein- 0.5g

Ingredients

- 1 large free-range egg yolk
- 1 tsp. Dijon mustard
- 285ml extra virgin olive oil
- 285ml olive oil
- ½ small clove garlic, peeled
- Lemon juice, to taste
- Freshly ground black pepper
- 1 tsp. Sea salt, plus more to season

Directions

1. Using mortar and pestle, mash up the garlic together with a teaspoon of salt.

2. Put the yolk and mustard in a bowl and whisk them together. Gradually add the oils little by little. Once you've combined a quarter of the oils, you can proceed to add larger amounts.

3. Once the mixture thickens, add the lemon juice and when all the oils have been incorporated, add the garlic-salt mixture. Season with salt and pepper.

Caramel Sauce

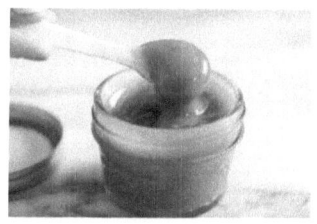

Servings: 10
Nutritional Information: Calories- 42; Fats- 0g; Carbohydrates- 10g; Protein- 0g

Ingredients

- 2/3 cup raw, organic milk
- 1/3 cup coconut palm sugar
- 1 tbsp. cornstarch
- 2 tsp. pure vanilla extract
- A dash of kosher or sea salt

Directions

1. Combine milk, cornstarch, sugar, and salt in a medium saucepan. Place over medium heat and cook until you achieve your desired thickness or consistency. Remove the pan from the heat and stir in the vanilla extract.

2. Refrigerate unused sauce. You can reheat it over low heat by the time you want to use it again. If it becomes too thick after refrigeration, you can add milk during reheating process.

Clean Eating Peanut Butter

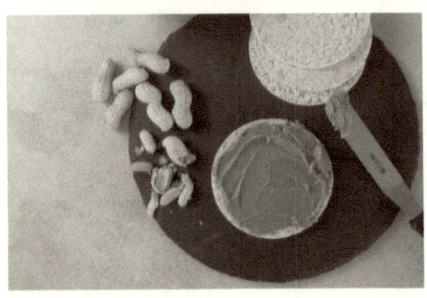

Servings: 12-14
Nutritional Information (per 2 tablespoons): Calories-166; Fats-14.4g; Carbohydrates- 4.7g; Protein- 7.5g

Ingredients

- 3 cups shelled raw peanuts
- ½ tsp. sea salt

Directions

1. Preheat the oven to 350°. Spread the peanuts on a baking sheet and roast them for approximately 20 minutes, stirring halfway through to avoid burning them. Let them cool for about 10 minutes.

2. Transfer the peanuts to a food processor or blender with plunger attachment. Season them with salt and process for 5-10 minutes or until you achieve a smooth and creamy consistency. Transfer the peanut butter into a sterilized jar and refrigerate.

Garlic-Parmesan Popcorn

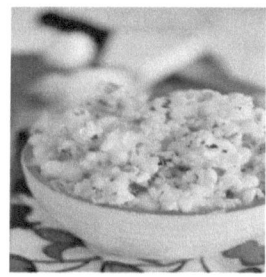

Servings: 5
Nutritional Information: Calories-73; Fats- 4g; Carbohydrates- 7g; Protein- 2g

Ingredients

- 1 cup popcorn kernels
- ½ cup Parmesan, freshly and finely grated
- 3 tbsp. unsalted butter
- 2 cloves garlic, minced
- 2 tbsp. vegetable oil
- ½ tsp. cayenne pepper
- Salt

Directions

1. Place a small saucepan over medium heat and melt the butter. Add the garlic and cook for a minute, stirring constantly. Remove the pan from the heat and set aside to cool.

2. Set a deep pot (this should have a tight-fitting lid) over high heat. Heat oil and add the kernels. Cover with a lid and cook for 1 minute.

3. Shake the pot in a back-and-forth motion over the burner until the kernels start to pop.

4. Continue to cook, shaking the pot in the process, for about 5 minutes or until the popping subsides. Remove the pot from the heat and transfer the popcorn to a large bowl.

5. Put butter-garlic mixture and sprinkle with parmesan and cayenne. Carefully toss the popcorn and season with salt. Store in an airtight container or resealable bags and refrigerate.

Homemade Cherry Pie Bars

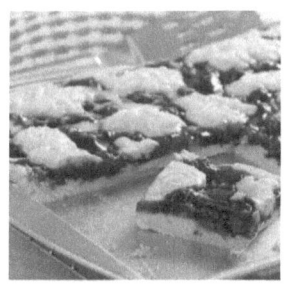

Servings: 18
Nutritional Information: Calories-200; Fats- 8g; Carbohydrates- 28g; Protein- 4g

Ingredients

- 8-10 Medjool dates, pitted
- 1 ½ cups raw almonds
- 1 ½ cups dried cherries
- Water

Directions

1. Combine all ingredients in a food processor. Gradually add water until you see the mixture gather together. Get an 8x8-inch glass baking dish and line it with parchment paper. Allow some paper to stick out the sides.

2. Press the mixture into the baking dish and refrigerate to make it firm. When the mixture has firmed up, cut it into bars using a pizza cutter.

Quince Crumble Bars

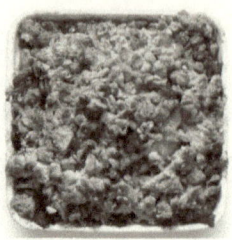

Servings: 12
Nutritional Information: Calories-1320; Fats- 37g; Carbohydrates-247g; Protein- 7g

Ingredients

- 900g quinces, washed and dried
- 250g compote (quince)
- 175g salted butter, chilled and cut into pieces
- 500g raw sugar
- 90g granulated sugar
- 4 tbsp. granulated sugar
- 250g flour
- Ground nutmeg
- Ground cinnamon
- 1 tbsp. Marsala wine
- Lemon juice

Directions

1. To prepare the quince compote, peel it. Also, remove the core and seeds. Cut into wedges and put them in a deep saucepan. Drizzle them with the juice of 1 lemon so they won't brown. Add a cup of water and simmer for 15 minutes.

2. Once done, drain and transfer into a blender to puree the quince. Put the puree back into the saucepan, add sugar, and

bring it to a boil. Let it simmer for 20 minutes, stirring frequently.

3. Pour the mixture in a 2-centimeter deep baking dish and spread it using a spatula. Cover with plastic wrap and let it rest for 3 days in a cool, dry place. After 3 days, cut the compote into squares using a wet knife. Sprinkle the bars with sugar before storing them in a metal canister.

4. Next, to prepare the quince crumble bars, line an 18x18-centimeter baking dish with wax paper.

5. To prepare the quince crumble bars, line a baking dish measuring 18x18 centimeters with wax paper.
6. In a mixing bowl, incorporate the sugar, flour, Marsala, and flour. Add the chilled butter and mix using your hands. The consistency must resemble that of an oatmeal.

7. Put ¾ of the mixture in the baking dish and press. Spread the compote over the mixture and top it with the remaining ¼ mixture. Bake at 350° for about 45 minutes. Remove from the oven and let it cool completely before cutting it into bars.

Pumpkin Candied Popcorn

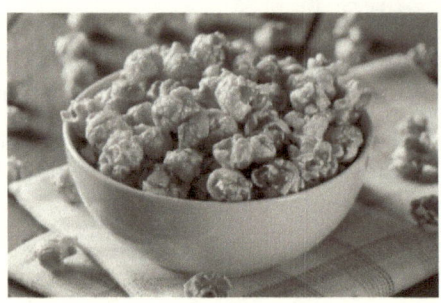

Servings: 5
Nutritional Information: Calories- 130; Fats- 7g; Carbohydrates- 18g; Protein- 1g

Ingredients

- ¼ cup popped popcorn kernels
- 1 tsp. coconut oil
- ¼ cup pumpkin
- ¼ cup brown rice syrup
- ¼ cup honey
- 3/4 tsp. homemade pumpkin spice (see recipe)

Directions

1. In a large pot, pop the popcorn kernels in 1 tsp. coconut oil. Get rid of the un-popped ones. In a small saucepan, incorporate all other ingredients and cook. Stir well as you bring it to a gentle boil. Make sure that the pumpkin is completely dissolved. Do not leave any lumps.

2. Pour the sauce over the popcorn and mix until everything is coated. Let the pot cool and put it in the fridge for about 3 hours. You can transfer the popcorn in an airtight container for up to 2 weeks.

Clean Eating Pumpkin Pie Spice

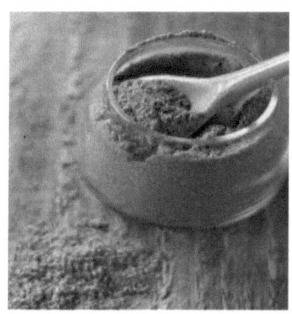

Servings: 5
Nutritional Information (per tablespoon): Calories-19.2; Fats- 0.7g; Carbohydrates- 3.9g; Protein- 0.3g

Ingredients

- 1 tbsp. ground allspice
- 2 tbsp. ground ginger
- 6 tbsp. ground cinnamon
- 1 tsp. ground nutmeg
- 2 tsp. ground cloves

Directions

1. Simply combine them well. Store in an airtight spice jar for up to 8 months.

Clean Eating Breakfast Cookies

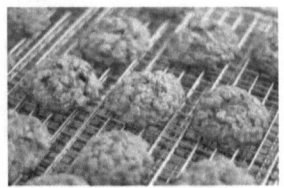

Servings: 12-14
Nutritional Information: Calories- 279; Fats- 17g; Carbohydrates- 29g; Protein- 7g

Ingredients

- 2 ripe bananas, mashed
- ¾ cup peanut butter
- 1 cup quick oats
- 1 cup old-fashioned oats
- ¾ cup dried fruit or raisins
- ½ cup unsalted cashew nuts
- ½ cup sunflower seeds
- ¼ cup ground flax
- ¼ cup honey, warmed
- ¼ cup coconut oil, melted
- 1 tsp. ground cinnamon
- ½ tsp. sea salt

Directions

1. Preheat oven to 325°. In a medium bowl, mix the honey, peanut butter, and coconut oil until you achieve a smooth consistency.

2. In a large bowl, put all the remaining ingredients together. Add the peanut butter mixture and stir well. Prepare a cooking sheet lined with wax paper. Drop about ¼ cup- sized scoops and

carefully spread to flatten. Bake for about 15 minutes or until the edges turn lightly browned.

3. Remove from the oven and let it cool completely before storing them in an air-tight container. You can freeze them for up to 6 months.

Apple Peanut Butter Sandwich

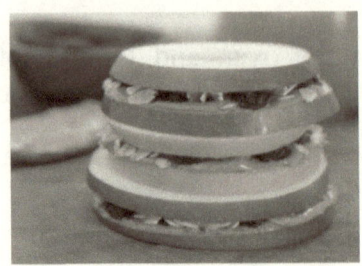

Servings: 5
Nutritional Information: Calories-203; Fats- 10g; Carbohydrates- 22g; Protein- 5g

Ingredients

- 10 thick apple slices, core removed
- 5 tbsp. peanut butter
- 5 tbsp. raisins
- 2 ½ tbsp. unsweetened coconut
- Lemon juice

Directions

1. Brush lemon juice on both sides of apple slices to avoid browning. Spread peanut butter on one apple slice.

2. Add the raisins and coconut. Top with another slice. Store in an airtight container and refrigerate.

Honey Nut Granola

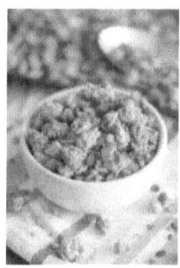

Servings: 16
Nutritional Information: Calories- 152; Fats- 4g; Carbohydrates- 26g; Protein- 7g

Ingredients

- 3 cups rolled oats
- 1 cup sliced almonds
- ¾ cup honey
- ½ tsp. pure almond extract
- 1 tsp. pure vanilla extract
- 1 tsp. cinnamon
- 2 tbsp. light or dark brown sugar
- ¼ tsp. salt

Directions

1. Preheat oven to 325°. In a large bowl, incorporate the oats, brown sugar, cinnamon, almonds, and salt.

2. In a small bowl or measuring cup, mix the almond extract, honey, and vanilla.

3. Put the honey mixture into the oat mixture and stir well. Make sure that everything is well coated. You can use a spoon or your clean hands.

4. Prepare a baking sheet by coating it with cooking spray. Spread the mixture on an even layer.

5. Bake 25-30 minutes or until it's golden brown. Remember to stir every 7-10 minutes. Keep an eye on it as granola can burn easily. Remove from oven and let it cool completely before storing in an airtight container.

Buffalo Hummus

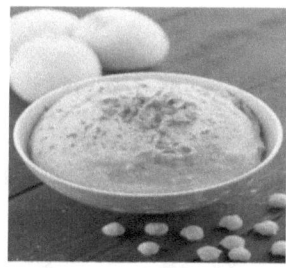

Servings: 10
Nutritional Information: Calories- 114; Fats- 5g; Carbohydrates- 15g; Protein- 5g

Ingredients

- 2 cans chickpeas, drained
- ¼ cup raw sesame seeds
- 1 clove garlic
- 1 tbsp. olive oil
- Juice from half of a lemon
- 2-3 tbsp. hot sauce
- ¼ cup crumbled blue cheese
- 1-2 tsp. of water

Directions

1. Put all the ingredients into a blender in order as listed above and secure lid. Process the ingredients on high for 1-2 minutes or until you achieve your desired texture. Add water to adjust the consistency. Store in an airtight container and refrigerate for up to a week.

Healthy Energy Bites

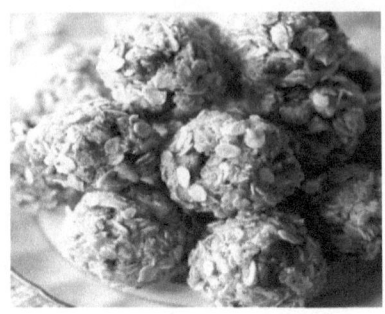

Serving: 10
Nutritional Information: Calories- 94; Fats- 5.5g; Carbohydrates- 10g; Protein- 2.5g

Ingredients

- 1 cup rolled oats
- ⅓ cup honey
- ½ cup almond butter
- ½ cup chocolate chips
- ½ cup ground flax seeds
- 1 tsp. vanilla

Directions

1. In a mixing bowl, combine all the ingredients. Make little balls and arrange them on a cookie sheet lined with parchment. Put in an airtight container and refrigerate.

Mayonnaise-less Avocado & Greek Yogurt Tuna Salad

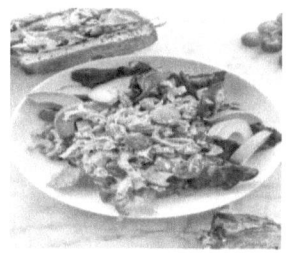

Servings: 5
Nutritional Information: Calories- 117; Fats- 4g; Carbohydrates- 4g; Protein- 18g

Ingredients

- 1 ripe avocado
- 2 x 4 oz. can high-quality tuna fish
- ¼ cup plain Greek yogurt
- ½ tsp. granulated garlic
- 1 celery stalk, chopped
- ½ tsp. onion powder
- 1 tbsp. dill relish
- ½ red onion, chopped
- Juice from ½ of a lemon
- ¼ tsp. black ground pepper
- ¼ tsp. salt

Directions

1. In a medium mixing bowl, mash the avocado and combine with the Greek yogurt. Mix until you achieve a smooth consistency.

2. Add the onion powder, dill relish, granulated garlic, pepper, and salt. Mix well to incorporate everything. Add the tuna, celery, and red onion and stir well.

3. Add the juice of lemon and stir again. Transfer in an airtight plastic or glass container and refrigerate. Serve with crackers or vegetables on the side. You can also serve this on a sandwich.

Pumpkin Spice Overnight Oats

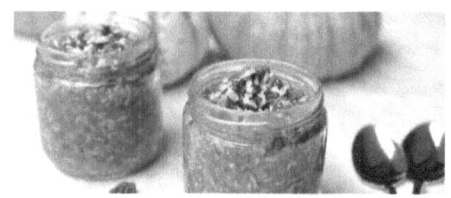

Servings: 5 jars
Nutritional Information: Calories- 254; Fats- 8g; Carbohydrates- 41g; Protein- 7g

Ingredients

- 2 ½ cup unsweetened coconut milk
- 2 ½ cup old fashioned oats
- 10 tbsp. pumpkin puree
- 10 tsp. pure maple syrup
- 5 tsp. walnuts, chopped
- 5 tsp. ground flaxseed
- 1 ¼ tsp. pumpkin pie spice
- 1 ¼ tsp. vanilla extract

Directions

1. Combine oats, coconut milk, flaxseed, pumpkin puree, maple syrup, vanilla extract, and pumpkin pie spice in a pint-size mason jar.

2. Stir well until the ingredients are completely incorporated. Place the lid and refrigerate for up to 5 days.

Conclusion

One can find meal prepping, a convenient, and cost-effective way of preparing your food. Instead of waking up early every time to prepare breakfast as well as cook for dinnertime after a hard day's work, you can easily pull out your ready-made meals anytime and enjoy eating a healthy clean meal.

This will not only be convenient but will likewise teach you how to organize your meals without the hassles of planning and cooking every day. You can organize everything from purchasing your kitchen supplies, containers, storage facilities, and more than everything – your time which is a valuable commodity.

The more time you save for all these, the more time you can spend on other tasks. Knowing that meal preparation and cooking activities are tedious and time-consuming, with the meal prep, you can just buy supplies in bulk, cook once or twice a week, and then you can enjoy the whole week free from kitchen stress.

With the prepared meal plan included in this book, you can now have a template for your 10-week diet plan without going through the usual time-consuming planning method. Feel free to change your meal recipes or incorporate them into your own weekly plans. Remember that all recipes included here are all clean food, assuring you of well-balanced and heathier meals for you and your family.

Final Words

I would like to thank you for downloading my book and I hope I have been able to help you and educate you about something new.

If you have enjoyed this book and would like to share your positive thoughts, could you please take 30 seconds of your time to go back and give me a review on my Amazon book page!

I greatly appreciate seeing these reviews because it helps me share my hard work!

Again, thank you and I wish you all the best with your cooking journey!

Last Chance to Get YOUR Bonus!

FOR A LIMITED TIME ONLY – Get Olivia's best-selling book *"The #1 Cookbook: Over 170+ of the Most Popular Recipes Across 7 Different Cuisines!"* absolutely FREE!

Readers have absolutely loved this book because of the wide variety of recipes. It is highly recommended you check these recipes out and see what you can add to your home menu!

Once again, as a big thank-you for downloading this book, I'd like to offer it to you *100% FREE for a LIMITED TIME ONLY!*

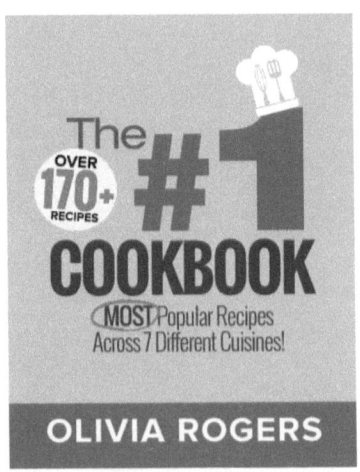

Get your free copy at:

TheMenuAtHome.com/Bonus

Disclaimer

This book and related site provides recipe and food advice in an informative and educational manner only, with information that is general in nature and that is not specific to you, the reader. The contents of this book and related site are intended to assist you and other readers in your personal efforts. Consult your physician or nutritionist regarding the applicability of any information provided in our information to you.

Nothing in this book should be construed as personal advice or diagnosis, and must not be used in this manner. The information provided about conditions is general in nature. This information does not cover all possible uses, actions, precautions, side-effects, or interactions of medicines, or medical procedures. The information in this site should not be considered as complete and does not cover all diseases, ailments, physical conditions, or their treatment.

No Warranties: The authors and publishers don't guarantee or warrant the quality, accuracy, completeness, timeliness, appropriateness or suitability of the information in this book, or of any product or services referenced by this site.

The information in this site is provided on an "as is" basis and the authors and publishers make no representations or warranties of any kind with respect to this information. This site may contain inaccuracies, typographical errors, or other errors.

Liability Disclaimer: The publishers, authors, and other parties involved in the creation, production, provision of information, or delivery of this site specifically disclaim any responsibility, and shall not be held liable for any damages, claims, injuries, losses, liabilities, costs, or obligations including any direct, indirect, special, incidental, or consequences damages (collectively known as "Damages") whatsoever and howsoever caused, arising out of, or in connection with the use or misuse of the site and the information contained within it, whether such Damages arise in contract, tort, negligence, equity, statute law, or by way of other legal theory.

www.ingramcontent.com/pod-product-compliance
Lightning Source LLC
Chambersburg PA
CBHW031123080526
44587CB00011B/1088